MRCP PART I
MCQ REVISION BOOK

MRCP PART I
MCQ REVISION BOOK

Compiled and edited by
PHILIP A. KALRA, MA MB BCHIR MRCP
Senior registrar in general medicine and nephrology
Royal Preston, Manchester Royal and Hope Hospitals
in collaboration with staff from the Manchester teaching hospitals.

MCQ Examination Technique by
JOHN ANDERSON, MB BS FRCP
Regional Postgraduate Dean and Professor of
Medical Education,
University of Newcastle- upon-Tyne.

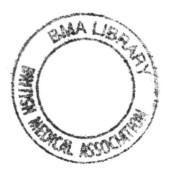

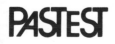

PASTEST

First Published 1981
Second Edition 1985
Reprinted 1987, 1989
Third Edition 1992
Reprinted 1993, 1995, 1997

ISBN 0 906896 86X

A catalogue record for this book is available from the British Library.

Text prepared by Turner Associates, Congleton, Cheshire.
Printed by BPC Wheatons, Exeter.

CONTENTS

Brackets indicate the number of questions in each section.

PREFACE

In this third edition of PasTest multiple choice questions for the MRCP Part I, we have made several alterations to the last edition, published in 1985.

The book has been extensively revised and approximately 40% of the questions and explanations are completely new. We have carefully observed the question content of the Royal College examinations over the last few years, and the book accordingly attempts to reproduce the format and the content of the actual MRCP Part I examination.

The emphasis on basic science questions has been continued, but more are now to be found within the relevant individual subject sections. As before, the section on statistics has a disproportionate number of questions, as does the section on GU medicine and AIDS in order to cover the rapid expansion of knowledge within this latter specialty. In addition we have included a comprehensive section discussing examination technique and a revision checklist of common question topics seen in the official examination. The subject content of an average examination is also highlighted.

You may well find that some of the questions are more difficult than those seen in the College examination; this is deliberate, and we have tried to select questions covering subjects that many candidates find particularly taxing. It is hoped that with the detailed teaching notes and cross-referencing provided this book will prove to be an invaluable aid to revision.

My thanks are due to many colleagues from the Manchester teaching hospitals for their help and co-operation in the preparation of this book, and I would especially like to thank Mrs Freydis Campbell for her considerable help and enthusiasm throughout the project.

PA Kalra

PasTest Intensive Courses for MRCP Part 1

PasTest Intensive Revision Courses for MRCP Part 1 (adult medicine or paediatrics) are designed for candidates who wish to pass first time. These officially approved six day courses are held in January, June and September in London, Manchester, Bristol and Stirling. Past exam questions and favourite MRCP topics are discussed and analysed together with advice on exam technique. High quality teaching notes and practice exams are included. The pass rate for candidates who have attended PasTest courses is excellent.

For full details contact:

PasTest, Freepost, Knutsford, Cheshire WA16 7BR
Tel: 01565 755226   Fax: 01565 650264.

MCQ EXAMINATION TECHNIQUE

Multiple Choice Questions are the most reliable, reproducible and internally consistent method we have of testing recall of factual knowledge. Yet there is evidence that they are able to test more than simple factual recall; reasoning ability and an understanding of basic facts, principles and concepts can also be assessed. A good MCQ paper will discriminate accurately between candidates on the basis of their knowledge of the topics being tested. It must be emphasised that the most important function of an MCQ paper of the type used in the MRCP Part I, is to rank candidates accurately and fairly according to their performance in that paper. Accurate ranking is the key phrase; this means that all MCQ examinations of this type are, in a sense, competitive. The majority of candidates achieve very similar scores near to the cut off point and an extra two or three marks may be all you need to push your score into the pass bracket. You therefore need to improve your exam technique to be sure of getting every mark you possibly can. The Part I pass rate is set at 35%, and so the pass mark varies, but it is usually around 55-60%.

Examination Technique.

The safest way to pass Part I MRCP is to know the answers to all of the questions, but it is equally important to be able to transfer this knowledge accurately onto the answer sheet. All too often, candidates suffer through an inability to organise their time, through failure to read the instructions carefully or through failure to read and understand the questions. First of all you must allocate your time with care. There are 60 questions to complete in 2½hours; this means 2½ minutes per question or 10 questions in 25 minutes. Make sure that you are getting through the exam at least at this pace, or, if possible, a little quicker, thus allowing time at the end for revision and a re-think on some of the items that you have deferred.

You must read the question (both stem and items) carefully. You should be quite clear that you know what you are being asked to do. Once you know this, you should indicate your responses by marking the paper boldly, correctly and clearly. Take care not to mark the wrong boxes and think very carefully before making a mark on the answer sheet. Regard each item as being independent of every other item – each refers to a specific quantum of knowledge. The item (or the stem and the item taken together) make up a statement. You are required to indicate whether you regard this statement as 'True' or 'False' and you are also able to indicate 'Don't know'. Look only at a single statement when answering –disregard all the other statements presented in the question. They have nothing to do with the item you are concentrating on.

Marking your answer sheets.

The answer sheet will be read by an automatic document reader, which transfers the information it reads to a computer. It must therefore be filled out in accordance with the instructions. A sample of the answer sheet, together with the instructions, is printed in the booklet of Examination Regulations available from the Royal College. Study these instructions carefully, well before the exams; the invigilators will also draw your attention to them at the time of the examination. You must first fill in your name on the answer sheet, and then fill in your examination number. It is critical that this is filled in correctly.

As you go through the questions, you can either mark your answers immediately on the answer sheet, or you can mark them in the question book first of all, transferring them to the answer sheets at the end. If you adopt the second approach, you must take great care not to run out of time, since you will not be allowed extra time to transfer marks to the answer sheet from the question book. The answer sheet must always be marked neatly and carefully according to the instructions given. Careless marking is probably one of the commonest causes of rejection of answer sheets by the document reader. For although the computer operators will do their best to interpret correctly the answer you intended, and will then correct the sheet accordingly, the procedure introduces a possible new source of error. You are, of course, at liberty to change your mind by erasing your original selection and selecting a new one. In this event, your erasure should be carefully, neatly, and completely carried out.

Try to leave time to go over your answers again before the end, in particular going back over any difficult questions that you wish to think about in more detail. At the same time, you can check that you have marked the answer sheet correctly. However, repeated review of your answers may in the end be counter-productive, since answers that you were originally confident were absolutely correct, often look rather less convincing at a second, third or fourth perusal. In this situation, first thoughts are usually best and too critical a revision might lead you into a state of confusion.

To guess or not to guess.

Do not mark at random. Candidates are frequently uncertain whether or not to guess the answer. However, a clear distinction must be made between a genuine guess (i.e. tails for True, heads for False) and a process of reasoning by which you attempt to work out an answer that is not immediately apparent by using first principles and drawing on your knowledge and experience. Genuine guesses should not be made. You might be lucky, but if you are totally ignorant of the answer, there is an equal chance you will be wrong and with the negative marking system you will thus lose marks. This is not a chance that is worth taking, and you should not hesitate to state 'Don't know' if this genuinely and honestly expresses your view.

Although you should not guess, you should not give in too easily. What you are doing is to increase, as much as possible, the odds that the answer you are going to give is the correct one, even though you are not 100% certain that this is the case. Take time to think, therefore, drawing on first principles and reasoning power, and delving into your memory stores. Do not, however, spend an inordinate amount of time on a single item that is puzzling you. Leave it, and, if you have time, return to it. If you are 'fairly certain' that you know the right answer or have been able to work it out, it is reasonable to mark the answer sheet accordingly. There is a difference between being 'fairly certain' (odds better than 50:50 that you are right) and totally ignorant (where any response would be a guess). The phrase 'MCQ technique' is often mentioned, and is usually used to refer specifically to this question of 'guessing' and 'Don't know'. Careful thought and reasoning ability, as well as honesty, are all involved in so-called 'technique', but the best way to increase the odds that you know the right answers to the questions is to have a sound basic knowledge of medicine and its specialties.

Trust the examiners.
Do try to trust the Examiners. Accept each question at its face value, and do not look for hidden meanings, catches and ambiguities. Multiple Choice Questions are not designed to trick or confuse you, they are designed to test your knowledge of medicine. Don't look for problems that aren't there – the obvious meaning of a statement is the correct one and the one that you should read.

Candidates often try to calculate their scores as they go through the paper; their theory is that if they reach a certain score they should then be safe in indicating 'Don't know' for any items that they have left blank without needing to take the trouble to think out answers. This approach is not to be recommended. No candidate can be certain what score he or she will need to achieve a pass in the examination, and everyone will overestimate the score they think they have obtained by answering questions confidently. The best approach is to answer every question honestly and to make every possible effort to work out the answers to more difficult questions, leaving the 'Don't know' option to indicate exactly what it means. In other words, your aim should always be to obtain the highest possible score on the MCQ paper.

To repeat the five most important points of technique
1. Read the question carefully and be sure you understand it.
2. Mark your responses clearly, correctly and accurately.
3. Use reasoning to work out answers, but if you do not know the answer and cannot work it out, indicate 'Don't know'.
4. Be bold and 'play your hunches'. If you are *reasonably* certain that you know the right answer, respond accordingly. Don't confine your answers only to those of which you are absolutely certain.
5. The best way to obtain a good mark is to have as wide a knowledge as possible of the topics being tested in the examination.

J.A.

POPULAR TOPICS FOR THE MRCP I EXAM

Cardiology
Wave form of JVP
Arrhythmias
ASD
Cardiovascular physiology
Constrictive pericarditis
Infective endocarditis
Mitral stenosis
Pulmonary embolus
Ventricular septal defect

Endocrinology
Acromegaly
Aldosterone secretion/action
Cushing's syndrome
Diabetes
Hypercalcaemia
Hyperlipidaemia
Hypothyroidism
Polydipsia
Thyrotoxicosis

Gastroenterology
Coeliac disease/malabsorption
Crohn's disease
Diarrhoea
Haemochromatosis
Hepatitis
Motility disorders
Primary biliary cirrhosis
Ulcerative colitis
Wilson's disease

Genetics
Autosomal dominant conditions
Autosomal recessive conditions
Sex-linked disorders

Haematology
Anaemia
Folate/iron deficiency
Haemolytic anaemias

Haemophilia
Hodgkin's lymphoma
Myeloma
Polycythaemia rubra vera
Sickle cell disease
Thalassaemia

Infectious diseases
AIDS
Amoebiasis
Chlamydial disease
Hepatitis B
Infectious mononucleosis
Insect bite transmission
Leptospirosis
Malaria
Syphilis

Metabolic disorders
Osteoporosis
Paget's disease
Porphyria
Rickets

Neurology
Alzheimers/dementia
Epilepsy
Facial nerve
Hereditary ataxias
Multiple sclerosis
Pupillary abnormality
Spinal cord lesions
Tremor
Ulnar, median, radial nerves

Nephrology and electrolyte disorders
Acute renal failure
Concentrated urine production
Goodpasture's syndrome
Hypokalaemia

Hyponatraemia
Immune complex deposition
Membranous glomerulonephritis
Minimal change/Nephrotic
  syndrome
Polycystic kidneys
Urinary abnormalities

Ophthalmology
Acute red eye
Cataract
Papilloedema
Visual field defects

Paediatrics
Cerebral palsy
Down's syndrome
Febrile convulsions
Neonatology/milestones
Nocturnal enuresis
Pertussis immunisation

Pharmacology
Drugs and renal or liver failure
Interactions with warfarin/
  phenytoin
Pairs of drugs contraindicated
  together
Porphyria and drugs

Psychiatry
Anorexia nervosa
Confusional state
Korsakoff syndrome

Manic depressive illness
Obsessional neurosis
Schizophrenia

Respiratory Medicine
Calcification on CXR
Emphysema
Haemoptysis
Occupational lung disease
Pneumonia
Pulmonary physiology
Sarcoidosis

Rheumatology
Ankylosing spondylitis
Behçet's disease
Digital gangrene/vasculitis
Gout
Reiter's syndrome
Rheumatoid arthritis
SLE

Statistics
Chi-squared
Clinical trials
Mean, mode and median
Normal distribution
Tests of significance

Toxicology
Aspirin overdose
Lead poisoning
Paracetamol overdose
Theophyline overdose

ACKNOWLEDGEMENTS

A sincere thank you is due to the many doctors in the Greater Manchester area whose contributions have made this book possible: William Brownlee, Alison Craig, Martin Davis, Peter Goulding, Elspeth Guthrie, Malcolm Littley, Chris Marguerie, Richard Motley (Cardiff), Zolf Mughal, Steve Owen and Jon Shaffer. We are most grateful to Dr Barry Hoffbrand of the Academic Centre, Whittington Hospital, London (editor of the second edition) for his invaluable advice and suggestions for this new edition.

INTRODUCTION

This book consists of 300 multiple choice questions the majority new and similar to those found in the MRCP Part I examination. Each question consists of an initial statement (or 'stem') followed by five possible completions (or 'items') identified by A B C D E. There is no restriction on the number of true or false items in a question. It is possible for all the items in a question to be true, or for all to be false.

The first 240 questions are divided into subjects and the last 60 form a complete practical exam. The subject breakdown corresponds to that of the official exam. The proportion of questions devoted to each subject also corresponds to that most likely to be found in the examination except that we have included additional questions on basic science and on statistics as explained in the Preface. You should bear in mind that our subject breakdown does not mean that only questions on these subjects will be asked, or that the proportion of questions devoted to each subject will remain the same. Questions on other subjects may occur in the examination and the proportions may vary.

Answers are given to every question together with teaching notes. For convenience, questions are printed on the right hand side of the page with the answers and explanations on the following page. This format is followed throughout, except for the 60 questions which form the Practice Exam where the answers and explanations are given at the end. The explanation for each question is necessarily brief; if you are well-informed you should find your memory adequately refreshed. If you are not, then you should seek further information from other sources. No references have been given as most students prefer to look up problem subjects in their favourite textbook.

To get the best value from this book your should arrive at an answer either 'True' or 'False' or 'Don't Know' for each item. Commit yourself before you look at the answer – this is really the best way to test your knowledge. In practice you can use the letters 'T', 'F' or 'D' to mark your answer against the question in the book. Alternatively you can prepare a grid on a separate piece of paper thus:-

	A	B	C	D	E
23					
24					

You can then mark your answers on the grid as you go along. To calculate your score give yourself $(+1)$ for each correct item, (-1) for each incorrect item and zero for each 'Don't Know' answer.

BASIC SCIENCES

1. **Prostaglandins**

   A are small molecular weight polypeptides
   B are chemically related to thromboxanes
   C are believed to act, in part, through stimulation of cyclic AMP accumulation
   D inhibit the secretion of renin
   E are produced in the seminal vesicles in man

2. **Plasma proteins**

   A migrate towards anode or cathode at different rates because of differences in electrical charges
   B are mostly in the form of cations
   C concentration falls early in starvation
   D are involved in the transportation of thyroid, adrenocortical, and gonadal hormones
   E are responsible for about 15% of the buffering capacity of the blood

3. **The effects of the following have been shown to be mediated by cyclic AMP:**

   A insulin
   B oxytocin
   C oestradiol
   D cortisol
   E parathyroid hormone

4. **The following statements about the orbit are correct:**

   A the trochlear (4th cranial) nerve supplies the inferior oblique muscle
   B the levator palpebrae superioris has a nerve supply from two different sources
   C the superior ophthalmic vein drains into the cavernous sinus
   D the ophthalmic artery is an end artery
   E the inferior rectus is supplied by the oculomotor (3rd cranial) nerve

Answers overleaf

1

1. **B C E**

   Prostaglandins are 20-carbon unsaturated fatty acids containing a cyclopentane ring. Thromboxanes, like prostaglandins, are formed from endoperoxides. They play an important role in platelet aggregation and local vasoconstriction these being of particular interest in the coronary and cerebral vessels. The chemically closely related prostacyclin is in contrast a vasodilator and inhibitor of platelet aggregation. Renal prostaglandins may stimulate secretion of renin.

2. **A D E**

   The different electrical charges of plasma proteins permit electrophoretic separation. They are mainly in the anion form, and contribute to the anion gap (see Q.148). Their weak ionization confers a buffering action. The main buffering action of plasma is provided by the carbonic acid – bicarbonate mechanism.

3. **B E**

   Most peptide hormones exert their effects through attachment to membrane bound receptors on target cells which in turn activate a rise in cyclic AMP concentration. Insulin is one exception to this rule, in which a different 'second messenger' system is involved. Steroid hormones are internalised and interact with nuclear receptors. Urinary cyclic AMP excretion is still occasionally used as a measure of parathyroid hormone action in the kidney.

4. **B C E**

   The abductor muscle (the lateral rectus) is supplied by the abducent (6th cranial) nerve and the superior oblique muscle is supplied by the trochlear (4th cranial) nerve. All the other muscles are supplied by the oculomotor (3rd cranial) nerve. The levator palpebrae superioris is supplied by the 3rd cranial and cervical sympathetic nerves and hence, paralysis may be due to lesions of either. The superior ophthalmic vein is one route by which infection can reach intracranial structures. The ophthalmic artery is one of the anastomotic links between the external carotid artery (via the facial artery) and the internal carotid artery from which it arises. Its branch to the retina is an end artery.

5. **The thyroid gland**

    A is closely related to the internal carotid artery
    B lies behind the parathyroid glands
    C normally weighs about 30 g
    D is closely related to the recurrent laryngeal nerve on the left only
    E embryological remnants may be found in the tongue at the junction of the anterior 2/3 and posterior 1/3.

6. **The foramen magnum transmits the**

    A basilar artery
    B hypoglossal nerves
    C pons
    D all of the spinal accessory nerve XI
    E posterior vertebral venous plexus

7. **On day 7 of the menstrual cycle as compared with day 21, there is**

    A a lower progesterone concentration
    B a lower body temperature
    C more developing follicles
    D a thicker endometrium
    E a fern-like pattern from a smear of cervical mucus

8. **Cholecystokinin-pancreozymin (CCK-PZ)**

    A is released from cells in the pancreatic ducts
    B is secreted in response to large amounts of circulating fatty acids
    C causes relaxation of the sphincter of Oddi
    D causes contraction of the gall bladder
    E acts synergistically with secretin

Answers overleaf

5. **C E**

The most important relations of the thyroid gland for physicians and surgeons are both recurrent laryngeal nerves, which lie postero-medially in the groove between the trachea and oesophagus, and the parathyroid glands which usually lie in close relation to the posterior border of the gland. The left recurrent laryngeal nerve is more exposed to disease because of its long course which starts in the superior mediastinum.

6. **D E**

The two vertebral arteries pass through the foramen magnum, only becoming the basilar artery on the pons lying superiorly. The hypoglossal nerves have their own canal (anterior condylar canal) lying just anterolaterally. The foramen magnum does, however, transmit all the cervical rootlets which ascend into the skull from upper cervical nerves, forming the spinal branch of the accessory nerve XI. All layers of the meninges, including contents of the extradural space, pass through the foramen.

7. **A B C E**

The first phase of the menstrual cycle, the follicular phase, is characterised by the development of the follicles. The progesterone concentration and hence, the body temperature, is lower than in the luteal phase of the cycle. Proliferation of the endometrium occurs in the second half of the cycle, and so the endometrium is relatively thinner on day 7. A cervical smear on day 7 gives a characteristic fern-like appearance.

8. **C D E**

CCK-PZ is produced by the intestinal mucosa. It is released following the ingestion of fat in a meal, but not necessarily by large amounts of circulating fatty acids. It aids in the digestion of fats by causing contraction of the gall bladder and relaxation of the sphincter of Oddi. It acts synergistically with secretin in the control of pancreatic secretion.

9. **The following statements concerning pulmonary stenosis are correct:**

    A   it is the commonest cardiovascular abnormality in Turner's syndrome
    B   the chest X-ray typically shows plethoric lung fields
    C   there is a recognised association with carcinoid syndrome
    D   an ejection click indicates that the stenosis is likely to be subvalvar
    E   the pulmonary component of the second sound is accentuated when the stenosis is severe

10. **The following conditions are recognised as predisposing to dissecting aneurysms of the aorta:**

    A   syphilitic aortitis
    B   rheumatic aortic valve disease
    C   Marfan's syndrome
    D   hypertension
    E   pregnancy

11. **The following statements about infective endocarditis are correct:**

    A   the most frequent manifestation of renal involvement is a nephrotic syndrome
    B   a common organism responsible for acute endocarditis is *Streptococcus faecalis*
    C   purpuric lesions are usually due to thrombocytopenia
    D   anti-nuclear factor is found in about 50% of cases
    E   the prognosis is worse with prolonged duration of symptoms

12. **In refractory heart failure**

    A   hyponatraemia is of prognostic significance
    B   Enalapril acts primarily by reducing venous return
    C   antacids are a potential hazard
    D   splenomegaly is a recognised finding
    E   blood urea levels rise in part due to overproduction of urea

Answers overleaf

9. C

Coarctation of the aorta is the commonest cardiovascular abnormality in Turner's syndrome (see Q.21). Pulmonary stenosis is common in Noonan syndrome, which is superficially similar. The chest X-ray is usually normal but may be oligaemic if the stenosis is severe, if there is right ventricular failure or right-to-left shunt. Carcinoid secretions of serotonin cause fibrous plaques, giving pulmonary stenosis and tricuspid regurgitation (see Q.24 practice exam). An ejection click points to valvular stenosis, as in aortic stenosis. With increasing severity the pulmonary component of the second sound becomes more delayed and softer, and the systolic murmur extends later into systole.

10. C D E

The factors that predispose to dissection are cystic medial necrosis, which occurs in Marfan's syndrome, and increased haemodynamic stress on the aorta as in hypertension, pregnancy and coarctation of the aorta.

11. E

The most frequently observed evidence of renal involvement in endocarditis is asymptomatic proteinuria and haematuria, caused by an immune-complex mediated focal proliferative glomerulo-nephritis which may also be associated with renal failure and nephrotic syndrome. *S. faecalis* is a common cause of subacute endocarditis, whilst *Staphylococcus aureus* and *Strep. pneumoniae* are commonly responsible for the acute form of the disease. Petechiae occur in the skin, retina and under the nails, and are probably due to immunological changes. Such changes account for low serum complement levels and positive rheumatoid factor tests, but ANF is not found (see Q.145). Thrombocytopenia is rare. Treatment started within two weeks after onset of symptoms gives a 90% survival. If treatment is delayed longer than eight weeks survival drops to 74%.

12. A C D E

Hyponatraemia is often due to diuretic therapy but occurs especially with advanced disease. Of the vasodilators used for heart failure, enalapril (an ACE inhibitor) acts primarily on arteries, nitrates on veins and nitroprusside and prazosin on both sides of the circulation. Some antacids, such as magnesium trisilicate mixture, contain substantial amounts of sodium chloride. Splenomegaly occurs with long-standing liver congestion usually associated with tricuspid regurgitation. Heart failure is a catabolic process with tissue breakdown contributing to uraemia and to cardiac cachexia.

13. **Characteristic features of the mitral valve prolapse (floppy mitral valve) syndrome include**

    A   early systolic murmur at apex
    B   mid-systolic click
    C   a liability to infective endocarditis
    D   a poor prognosis
    E   a higher incidence in males

14. **The following statements concerning exercise testing in heart disease are correct:**

    A   a normal exercise test excludes significant ischaemic heart disease
    B   excrcise testing is a useful way of assessing the severity of aortic stenosis in adults
    C   exercise testing may reveal significant arrhythmias
    D   digoxin therapy may cause difficulty in interpreting the ECG changes occurring with exercise
    E   a fall in the systolic blood pressure by 20 mm Hg or more during exercise suggests that severe coronary artery disease may be present

15. **The following statements about atrial flutter are correct:**

    A   the ventricular rate is characteristically about 150/min
    B   an irregular pulse is a recognised finding
    C   DC counter shock is a treatment of choice
    D   quinidine alone is a recognised treatment
    E   carotid sinus pressure is of value in diagnosis

16. **Recognised features of congestive (dilated) cardiomyopathy include**

    A   an increased risk of systemic embolism
    B   pansystolic murmurs
    C   asymmetrical hypertrophy of the intraventricular septum
    D   a history of alcoholism
    E   a family history of sudden death

Answers overleaf

13. B C

The characteristic murmur is ejection or late systolic. The murmur is often preceded by an ejection mid-systolic click. Liability to infective endocarditis relates to the amount of mitral reflux. The prognosis is generally good, although severe mitral regurgitation can occur requiring mitral valve replacements or repair. The condition was believed to be more common in females, but the sex incidence is now thought to be equal.

14. C D E

Both false positive and negative exercise tests occur but a normal test makes it unlikely that a major cardiac event will occur in the next year. Exercise testing is potentially hazardous in significant aortic valvular stenosis. This is also true for severe LV outflow tract obstruction due to hypertrophic cardiomyopathy. Exercise testing is useful in assessment of ventricular ectopic activity and in revealing ventricular tachycardia and atrial tachyarrhythmias. Any resting ST segment change, bundle branch block pattern or left ventricular hypertrophy makes interpretation of an exercise test difficult. A fall in blood pressure on exercise, (except if exercising soon after a myocardial infarction), suggests a poor prognosis.

15. A B C E

The atrial flutter rate ranges from 250 to 350/min, usually 300/min. In the untreated state there is usually 2:1 A-V block. The block may occasionally be variable, giving enough ventricular irregularity to simulate atrial fibrillation. The degree of A-V block can be increased by vagal stimulation (carotid sinus pressure) slowing the ventricular rate suddenly, and making the flutter waves more obvious in the ECG. Quinidine slows the flutter-rate and increases A-V conduction; the consequence in the absence of digitalis may be a 1:1 response and a dangerously rapid ventricular rate.

16. A B D

Congestive cardiomyopathy is characterized by a dilated heart with functional mitral and tricuspid regurgitation, and congestive heart failure. Emboli are common even in the absence of arrhythmias which also frequently complicate the picture. There are many causes of congestive cardiomyopathy including alcoholism, but a majority of cases in the UK are idiopathic, occurring in the middle-aged and elderly. Septal hypertrophy and familial sudden death are features of hypertrophic cardiomyopathy (HOCM) (see Q.5 practice exam).

17. The following statements about abdominal aortic aneurysms are correct:

A they typically arise above the renal arteries
B they are a recognised cause of ureteric obstruction
C cross-sectional ultrasound is the best way to detect and size the aneurysm
D the patient's prognosis is related to the size of the aneurysm
E a majority of cases present with rupture

18. The following are characteristic findings in constrictive pericarditis:

A atrial fibrillation
B normal heart size
C acute pulmonary oedema
D pulsus alternans
E third heart sound

19. The following are typical findings in acute rheumatic fever:

A apical rumbling presystolic murmur
B tender subcutaneous nodules
C cardiac conduction defects
D nail bed changes
E urticaria

20. Characteristic findings in complete atrio-ventricular (heart) block include

A variable intensity of the second heart sound
B increased ventricular rate after atropine
C collapsing brachial pulse
D regular giant 'a' waves in the jugular venous pulse
E beat to beat variation in the blood pressure

Answers overleaf

17. B C D

The majority of abdominal aortic aneurysms are atherosclerotic and arise below the renal arteries. Expansion may compress contiguous structures and cause ureteric obstruction (see Q.138). The majority of patients are asymptomatic at the time of diagnosis. Pain from the aneurysm usually means impending or actual rupture, which is more likely to occur in larger aneurysms; 50% of aneurysms with diameters greater than 6 cm rupture within one year.

18. A B E

Atrial fibrillation is present in about one third of cases. Cardiomegaly is often absent but when present is usually only moderate. The chest X-ray occasionally suggests considerable cardiomegaly due to gross thickening of the pericardium. Acute pulmonary oedema and pulsus alternans would suggest myocardial disease. The third heart sound of constrictive pericarditis (pericardial knock) represents rapid, but suddenly abbreviated, ventricular filling.

19. C

Significant murmurs indicating carditis are those of mitral and aortic regurgitation and an apical mid-diastolic rumbling murmur (Carey Coombs) which is often associated with mitral regurgitation. Mitral and aortic stenosis only develop after months or years. Rheumatic nodes are painless. The most frequent conduction defect is prolongation of the P-R interval. The classical cutaneous manifestation of rheumatic fever is erythema marginatum found mainly on the trunk and proximal parts of the limbs.

20. C E

A variable first heart sound occurs and is a sign of the asynchrony of atrial and ventricular contraction. This also gives rise to irregular giant 'a' ('cannon') waves. In acquired complete heart block the majority of cases have a pacemaker in the Purkinje system which responds poorly to exercise, vagal or sympathetic effects. In congenital heart block, the block and subsidiary pacemakers are higher and the ventricular response, particularly in the young, may be near normal. The arterial pulse has a wide pulse pressure with a large stroke volume and thus tends to feel collapsing. The volume of the blood pressure will vary with the atrial contribution (see also Q.6 practice exam).

21. Coarctation of the thoracic aorta

    A is a predominantly female disease

    B occurs characteristically proximal to the origin of the left subclavian artery

    C can give a continuous murmur

    D is associated with bicuspid aortic valves

    E has a good prognosis untreated after the age of twenty

22. In acute massive pulmonary embolism

    A clinical evidence of deep venous thrombosis is characteristically present

    B pulmonary embolectomy is the treatment of choice

    C the arterial pCO_2 is characteristically raised

    D the chest X-ray shows oligaemia in the lung fields in the majority of cases

    E subcutaneous heparin should be started immediately the diagnosis is suspected

23. The following statements about angina pectoris are correct:

    A it may occur with normal coronary arteries

    B it is associated with an abnormal resting ECG between attacks in about 90% of cases

    C it is typically worse later in the day

    D ST segment elevation on ECG is usual during an attack

    E it may be aggravated by lying down

24. Acute pericarditis is a recognised complication of

    A polyarteritis nodosa

    B gonorrhoea

    C thyrotoxicosis

    D amoebiasis

    E congestive cardiac failure

Answers overleaf

21. C D

Males outnumber females by more than 2:1. It is common in Turner's syndrome, which should be suspected in all females with coarctation. The commonest site for a coarctation is just distal to the left subclavian artery. If the lumen is very narrow, flow through it may occur throughout the cardiac cycle. The commonest cause of a diastolic murmur is, however, aortic regurgitation due to a bicuspid valve. Other associated malformations are PDA, VSD and mitral abnormalities. Left ventricular failure, cerebral haemorrhage, aortic dissection (see Q.10) and infective endocarditis are all serious hazards of untreated coarctation.

22. NONE CORRECT

The treatment of choice is intravenous thrombolysis and heparin; the subcutaneous route is only appropriate for prophylaxis. The arterial pCO_2 and pO_2 are characteristically reduced. The chest X-ray is normal more often than not but may show areas of radiolucency due to oligaemia. There may also be vessel 'cut off' and later, even without infarction, evidence of atelectasis. Diagnosis is best made by perfusion scanning, which also may be useful to monitor the effects of therapy (see also Q.26).

23. A E

Angina with normal coronary arteries is found in cardiomyopathies, severe aortic stenosis and pulmonary hypertension, as well as in otherwise normal hearts when coronary artery spasm or coronary blood flow abnormalities are implicated. The resting ECG is normal in 50% or more of patients between attacks. Many patients get angina on getting up in the morning and become symptom-free later in the day. ST segment elevation during an attack is the major feature of Prinzmetal's 'variant' angina. The mechanism of angina decubitus is unknown but this symptom usually indicates severe coronary disease.

24. A B D

Acute pericarditis is a recognised feature of all the connective tissue diseases and can complicate any septicaemia. It is a serious complication of amoebic abscesses of the left lobe of the liver (see Q.60 practice exam and Q.120). Although pericardial fluid accumulates in congestive cardiac failure, the amount is rarely significant and is not inflammatory.

25. In a patient with mitral stenosis in sinus rhythm, the following findings would indicate a severe lesion:

A long mid-diastolic murmur
B late, loud, opening snap
C soft first heart sound
D Graham-Steel murmur
E third heart sound

26. A dominant R wave in lead V1 of the ECG is a characteristic finding in

A acute pulmonary embolism
B Wolff-Parkinson-White syndrome
C left bundle branch block
D hyperkalaemia
E true posterior myocardial infarction

27. In ostium secundum atrial septal defect

A pregnancy is typically poorly tolerated
B a mid-diastolic murmur suggests a large shunt
C there is reversed splitting of the second heart sound
D atrial arrhythmias are an important feature
E the electrocardiograph shows left axis deviation

28. The following statements about the arterial pulse are correct:

A pulsus paradoxus is diagnostic of cardiac tamponade
B a bisferiens pulse suggests combined aortic stenosis and regurgitation
C pulsus alternans is a sign of impaired left ventricular function
D a slow rising carotid pulse is characteristic of severe mitral stenosis
E the femoral pulses are diminished but not delayed in coarctation of the aorta

Answers overleaf

25. A D

The intensity of the first heart sound and the opening snap reflects the mobility of the mitral valve leaflets and not the severity of the stenosis. In more severe mitral stenosis the LV pressure falls below that of the LA earlier in diastole, leading to an early opening snap and long diastolic murmur. The murmur of pulmonary regurgitation (Graham-Steel) occurs with severe pulmonary hypertension. A third heart sound indicates rapid filling of the left ventricle and this excludes severe mitral stenosis (unless it is a right ventricular sound, when there would be obvious signs of tricuspid regurgitation).

26. B E

Perhaps a majority of patients with acute pulmonary embolism show no ECG changes apart from sinus tachycardia and T-wave inversion over the right-sided precordial leads. $S_1Q_3T_3$ pattern, P pulmonale, right axis deviation and right bundle branch block occur, but a dominant R wave in V1 is not a feature of an acute load on the right side of the heart. This occurs, however, with right ventricular hypertrophy due to many causes as well as in WPW (type A) and true posterior myocardial infarcts (see also Q.22).

27. B D

This is the commonest type of ASD and may well present in adult life. Unless pulmonary hypertension is present pregnancy is well tolerated. A tricuspid mid-diastolic murmur indicates a large left-to-right shunt. This murmur, and the classical pulmonary area systolic murmur, lessen and disappear as pulmonary hypertension develops, and the shunt is reduced. Haemodynamic deterioration is often heralded by the onset of atrial fibrillation, flutter or tachycardia. Left axis deviation is the ECG hallmark of ostium primum ASD which involves the A-V valves.

28. B C

Pulsus paradoxus, a greater than the normal 10 mm Hg inspiratory decrease in systolic arterial pressure, occurs in cardiac tamponade, and, less commonly, in constrictive pericarditis. It is not diagnostic of pericardial disease, but occurs in cardiomyopathies, severe asthma, superior mediastinal obstruction and shock. A bisferiens pulse is also found in hypertrophic cardiomyopathy (see Q.5 practice exam) and pulsus alternans during or following paroxysmal tachycardia. Severe mitral stenosis gives a low pulse volume and coarctation a delayed femoral pulse, which may also be diminished in volume.

29. Concerning clinical trials

A phase II studies are usually conducted in healthy volunteers
B placebo drugs are physiologically inert
C the commonest criticism of negative trials is a type II error
D cross-over studies require fewer patients than group comparisons
E visual analogue scales are unreliable

30. Monitoring plasma concentrations is of value in the management of overdosage of

A propranolol
B lithium
C amitriptyline
D iron
E digoxin

31. In cardiopulmonary resuscitation

A witnessed asystole should be treated with IV calcium
B adrenaline improves cerebral blood flow
C atropine has no role in ventricular fibrillation
D modest acidosis is a contraindication to sodium bicarbonate
E intrabronchial route regimes require twice normal dosage

32. Thrombocytopenia is a recognised side effect of

A warfarin
B heparin
C gold
D bendrofluazide
E quinine

Answers overleaf

29. C D

The American FDA divides trials into 4 phases: I – first exposure in man, usually healthy volunteers; II – small comparative trials; III – large scale clinical trials; IV – post marketing surveillance. Placebos are pharmacologically inert (but physiologically active in up to 50% of subjects).

Most trials compare 2 groups but large numbers are required. Where this is not possible half the number of patients required are needed in a cross-over trial, the patients acting as their own 'control'. Cross-over studies produce order effects and carry-over effects and are only applicable if therapy modifies and does not cure the condition being treated. Reassessment should be objective if at all possible but subjective visual analogue scales are reliable. Type I errors (false positive) are less common than type II errors (false negative) as the main difficulty with many trials is inadequate numbers (see also Q.234 and Q.54 practice exam).

30. B D

Plasma monitoring is of prime value in the management of paracetamol and salicylate poisoning. It has a role with theophylline, barbiturates, iron and lithium. Tricyclic concentrations are difficult to measure and reflect toxicity poorly. Beta blocker and digoxin toxicity are better assessed by bioassay, i.e. pulse rate and cardiac output.

31. B C D E

Adrenaline, largely due to its alpha effect, is the first-choice drug for the different cardiac arrest dysrrhythmias. Atropine has a role in asystole; calcium should be reserved for electro-mechanical dissociation, hypocalcaemia and calcium antagonist overdosage. A pH >7.2 increases tissue oxygen uptake and bicarbonate should only be given if the pH is <7.1.

32. B C D E

Quinine, quinidine and heparin are the drugs most likely to produce thrombocytopenia. They induce production of platelet damaging antibodies. NSAIDs, gold and thiazides are a lesser risk, the mechanism being unclear. Chloramphenicol depresses platelet production.

33. The following are true statements concerning calcium channel blocking drugs:

   A diltiazem has no anti-arrhythmic properties
   B they dilate arteries more than veins
   C nifedipine increases pulse rate
   D verapamil is the most likely to cause constipation
   E verapamil is the least likely to produce heart failure

34. Recognised complications of vincristine therapy include the following:

   A diffuse pulmonary fibrosis
   B peripheral neuropathy
   C inappropriate ADH secretion
   D generalised pigmentation of the skin
   E paralytic ileus

35. The following drugs should be avoided in renal failure:

   A ampicillin
   B oxytetracycline
   C aluminium hydroxide
   D ferrous sulphate
   E nitrofurantoin

36. Aspirin potentiates the therapeutic action of the following:

   A warfarin
   B probenecid
   C indomethacin
   D diazepam
   E tetracyclines

Answers overleaf

33. B C D

There is much greater variability in this group of drugs than with e.g. beta blockers. Verapamil has the most potent anti-arrhythmic and negatively inotropic activity; dihydropipones like nifedipine are the most potent vasodilators with little direct effect on the heart. Diltiazem has a midway position between them.

34. B C E

Vincristine can cause neuropathy, joint pain, alopecia, paralytic ileus and inappropriate ADH secretion. Pulmonary fibrosis is seen with busulphan and bleomycin and skin pigmentation also occurs with busulphan.

Vincristine (Oncovin) is part of the MOPP regime for Hodgkin's disease, and is used in acute lymphoblastic leukaemia and other lymphomas.

35. B E

Tetracyclines, apart from doxycycline, should be avoided in renal failure as they are antianabolic, cause salt and water loss, raise the blood urea and can lead to permanent loss of nephrons. Nitrofurantoin is prone to give toxic levels and peripheral neuropathy in renal failure. It is also likely to be ineffective for urinary infections. Although aluminium hydroxide is used for phosphate lowering, there are concerns about aluminium retention with prolonged usage.

36. A C

Aspirin in large doses is hypoprothrombinaemic. In smaller doses, it increases the bleeding tendency by its antiplatelet and gastric irritant effects. Also, in large doses, aspirin is uricosuric, but in therapeutic doses of 1–2 g/day or less, it reduces urate excretion. Again, in large doses aspirin is hypoglycaemic (see also Q.26 practice exam).

37. **In chronic liver disease the following should be avoided:**

    A   digoxin
    B   pethidine
    C   paracetamol
    D   isoniazid
    E   imipramine

38. **The following drugs are contraindicated in breast feeding:**

    A   warfarin
    B   senna
    C   digoxin
    D   paracetamol
    E   cimetidine

39. **The blood brain barrier is rapidly permeable to**

    A   highly polar water-soluble drugs
    B   strong acids
    C   weak bases
    D   adrenaline
    E   amphetamine

40. **Patients with acute intermittent porphyria should avoid**

    A   alcohol
    B   rifampicin
    C   phenytoin
    D   aspirin
    E   oral contraceptives

Answers overleaf

37. **B D E**

The ability of the diseased liver to detoxify drugs is maintained to a considerable degree. Known hepatotoxins like some anti-TB drugs and phenothiazines should not be used. Drugs that are CNS depressants are likely to have increased efficacy and prolonged duration of action; antidepressants should also be avoided.

38. **B**

Most drugs enter breast milk by passive lipid diffusion. As the plasma drug concentration is relatively low compared to total body concentration, the load to a baby is small. Only drugs known to be toxic to the child, e.g. radio-iodine cytotoxics, should be avoided completely.

39. **C E**

The blood brain barrier is more easily soluble to lipid than to water soluble drugs. Highly polar drugs have lower concentrations of unionised molecules at pH 7.4 and penetrate slowly. The penetration of acid and basic drugs also depends on the lipid solubility of the unionised molecules. Adrenaline (acid) penetrates poorly but amphetamine (base) much more easily as it has fewer polar groups.

40. **A B C E**

Other drugs that should be avoided include sulphonamides, sulphonylureas, barbiturates and griseofulvin. These agents may precipitate acute porphyria by hepatic microsomal enzyme induction of ALA-synthetase, so stimulating the first step in the porphyrin synthetic pathway (see also Q.34 practice exam).

41. Thyroid function tests are affected by concomitant administration of

A phenytoin
B aspirin
C bromocriptine
D corticosteroids
E lithium

42. In paracetamol poisoning

A the earliest sign of hepatotoxicity is a raised alanine trans-
   aminase (ALT)
B patients established on cimetidine are at increased risk
C smokers are at decreased risk
D N-acetylcysteine is effective because it can donate -SH groups
E after recovery, future therapy with paracetamol is contra-
   indicated

43. The following are associated with cannabis abuse:

A irreversible reduction in academic performance
B persistent bradycardia
C hypotension
D hypertension
E status epilepticus

44. In theophylline overdosage

A plasma theophylline concentrations are a poor guide to toxicity
B convulsions indicate a bad prognosis
C hypokalaemia can be profound
D activated charcoal is ineffective
E centrally induced nausea and vomiting are poorly responsive to
   anti-emetics

Answers overleaf

41. A B C D E

Many drugs can affect thyroid function. Lithium iodides and amiodarone inhibit thyroxine secretion; phenytoin, salicylates, carbamazepine and corticosteroids increase thyroxine clearance and decrease plasma protein binding. Dopaminergic agents and corticosteroids suppress TSH.

42. D

Paracetamol toxicity after self-poisoning is the result of increased production of an alkylating metabolite. Enzyme inducers like tobacco increase metabolite production and hence toxicity whilst enzyme inhibitors like cimetidine have the reverse effect. The earliest sign of liver damage, and the most useful prognostic indicator, is the prothrombin time; values less than 100 seconds after 3–4 days are rarely associated with death. If recovery occurs it is complete.

43. C D

Chronic cannabis abuse produces reversible intellectual impairment. Initial reports of cerebral atrophy have not been confirmed. Cannabis smoke may be carcinogenic.

44. C E

The two major problems of serious overdosage are intractable vomiting and hypokalaemia; intravenous potassium supplementation may be required. Convulsions tend to occur after moderate/ severe overdosage and should be treated with repeated doses of diazepam. The most effective method of theophylline excretion is the use of repeated doses of activated charcoal after gastric lavage. Haemoperfusion should be reserved for patients unable to tolerate charcoal and for the seriously ill patient having severe acidosis, coma or circulatory instability in addition to a very high theophylline level.

45. The following are features of dermatitis herpetiformis:

A   a granular pattern of IgA antibodies at the dermo-epidermal junction of uninvolved skin
B   a rapid response to oral dapsone
C   gastrointestinal malabsorption
D   an increased incidence of malignancy
E   an association with HLA types B8, Dw3 and DRw3

46. The following conditions are more prevalent in immuno-compromised patients:

A   viral warts
B   Kaposi's sarcoma
C   squamous cell carcinomas
D   seborrhoeic dermatitis
E   scabies

47. Alopecia is a recognised feature of the following:

A   the treatment of psoriasis with etretinate
B   hyperthyroidism
C   lichen planus
D   severe illness
E   cyclosporin therapy

48. Purpuric skin lesions are a feature of

A   vitamin A deficiency
B   T cell lymphoma
C   corticosteroid therapy
D   pemphigus
E   pityriasis rosea

Answers overleaf

45. A B D E

The diagnosis of dermatitis herpetiformis is confirmed by the presence of IgA antibodies deposited in a granular pattern at the dermo-epidermal junction of uninvolved skin. A rapid response to dapsone is characteristic. Although most patients have a gluten-sensitive enteropathy, malabsorption is rare. There is an increased incidence of malignancy, particularly gastrointestinal lymphoma.

46. A B C D E

Transplant patients have an increased incidence of viral warts and squamous cell carcinoma as a result of long-term immuno-suppressive therapy. Kaposi's sarcoma is a characteristic finding in sexually transmitted HIV disease, although it is unusual in patients who acquired the condition through blood transfusion or intra-venous drug abuse, suggesting it may be due to a different infectious agent. Classical Kaposi's sarcoma occurs in Africans, European Jews and in people from the Po valley area of Italy. Seborrhoeic dermatitis is a feature of AIDS and may be due to overgrowth of pityrosporum yeast. Scabies infestation is more florid in the immunocompromised.

47. A C D

The retinoid drug, etretinate, is effective in a number of cutaneous disorders including psoriasis. It may cause a reversible hair loss. Lichen planus and discoid lupus erythematosus may cause scarring alopecia. Telogen effluvium occurs when a large number of hairs pass simultaneously into the telogen (or resting) phase. This may be precipitated by severe illness or childbirth and leads to these hairs being lost 2–3 months later. Cyclosporin may cause hypertrichosis.

48. B C

Perifollicular haemorrhages are a feature of vitamin C deficiency. Hypovitaminosis A presents with dry skin, follicular hyperkeratosis and xerophthalmia. T cell lymphoma may present with purpuric skin lesions. Both long term topical and systemic corticosteroid therapy may cause easy bruising and skin fragility.

49. Bullae are a feature of

A orf
B pompholyx eczema
C erythema nodosum
D pemphigoid
E erythema multiforme

50. Changes in the nail or adjacent tissue are seen in

A dermatomyositis
B psoriasis
C epidermolysis bullosa
D pyoderma gangrenosum
E following severe illness

51. Recognised causes of erythema nodosum include

A Behcet's disease
B sarcoidosis
C oral contraceptives
D preceding mycoplasmal infection
E diabetes mellitus

52. The following drugs are recognised causes of the rashes mentioned:

A captopril and lichenoid eruptions
B minocycline and skin pigmentation
C gold and exfoliative dermatitis
D aspirin and urticaria
E thiazides and photosensitivity

Answers overleaf

49. A B D E

Orf is a pox virus which causes a stomatitis in lambs and is transmitted to the hands of humans involved in their feeding. Eczema of the palms and soles usually develops large bullae hence the term 'pompholyx' (Greek for 'bubble'). Erythema nodosum does not develop bullae, but severe erythema multiforme may do. The bullae in pemphigoid are subepidermal and are more often intact than those in pemphigus which occur within the epidermis.

50. A B C E

Dilated capillaries around the distal nail fold are a feature of dermatomyositis. The nails in psoriasis show pitting and onycholysis. The nails may be deformed and lost in dystrophic forms of epidermolysis bullosa, although it is uncommon to see changes in the simple form of the disease.

Beau's lines are transverse grooves across the nail plate and result from altered growth during a period of severe illness.

51. A B C D

Erythema nodosum may be due to underlying systemic disease e.g. Crohn's disease, ulcerative colitis, Behcet's disease and sarcoidosis. It can be caused by various drugs, notably sulphonamides and oral contraceptives, and by preceding infection, especially streptococcal.

52. A B C D E

Virtually all drugs can cause cutaneous reactions. It is important to recognise that some drug-induced rashes may mimic specific types of skin disease. Lichen planus-like reactions may occur with gold, antimalarials, phenothiazines and captopril. Skin pigmentation may be induced by antimalarials, phenothiazines and minocycline. Oral contraceptives may produce chloasma. Exfoliative dermatitis may result from gold therapy. Aspirin may cause urticaria in patients with salicylate hypersensitivity, and can exacerbate idiopathic urticaria as a result of its pharmacological action. Thiazides, sulphonamides, tetracyclines and phenothiazines may cause a photosensitive rash.

53. In diabetic glomerulosclerosis

A arteriosclerosis is generally thought to play an important initiating role
B hypertension is usually the first clinical feature
C absence of diabetic retinopathy is exceptional
D nodular sclerosis (Kimmelsteil-Wilson lesion) is the commonest histological finding
E renal amyloid may be a late complication

54. In the treatment of non insulin dependent diabetes (NIDDM)

A hyperosmolar non-ketotic coma typically requires large doses of insulin
B insulin resistance contributes to the hyperglycaemia
C glibenclamide is safer than glipizide in the elderly
D metformin frequently causes hypoglycaemia
E chlorpropamide may cause facial flushing

55. The following are characteristically associated with hypoglycaemia:

A adrenocortical insufficiency
B retroperitoneal sarcoma
C alcohol intoxication
D multiple endocrine neoplasia Type 2a
E von Gierke's disease

56. In patients with phaeochromocytoma

A a tumour secreting adrenaline only is more likely to arise from a site other than the adrenals
B tumours in both adrenals occur in about ten per cent of cases
C preparation for surgery should generally start with a beta blocker drug
D hypercalcaemia is a recognised finding
E there is an association with follicular carcinoma of the thyroid

Answers overleaf

53. C
Mild proteinuria is the first clinical feature of diabetic glomerulo-sclerosis and is frequently associated with retinopathy and neuropathy. Hypertension often develops later and may exacerbate the condition, but amyloid is not a complication. Nodular sclerosis, although the most specific form of diabetic nephropathy, accounts for less than 20% of renal involvement.

54. B E
Despite the fact that insulin resistance is a major problem in the obese non-insulin dependent diabetic, patients presenting with hyper-osmolar coma are typically very sensitive to insulin. Small doses of insulin are therefore used initially to bring about slow changes in the disordered metabolic state. Although the half-life of glibenclamide is relatively short, it has active metabolites with a long half-life. Glipizide and its metabolites have a short duration of action and is therefore much safer in the elderly. Metformin does not normally induce clinical hypoglycaemia, even in overdose. Facial flushing with alcohol is an autosomal dominant determined condition present in 15–20% of patients treated with chlorpropamide.

55. A B C E
Hypoglycaemia is one of the characteristic biochemical findings in acute adrenal insufficiency (adrenal crisis); others include acidosis, hyperkalaemia, hyponatraemia and hypercalcaemia. Retroperitoneal tumours are always included in the differential diagnosis of spontaneous hypoglycaemia, as is an insulinoma, which may be a part of MEN type I (Pancreas, Pituitary, Parathyroid). Alcohol impairs hepatic glucose production and may precipitate hypo-glycaemia, particularly in otherwise well-controlled insulin-treated diabetics. Glycogen storage diseases that involve the liver (as in von Gierke's disease) may cause hypoglycaemia (see also Q.156).

56. B D
Extra-adrenal tumours lack the methylating enzyme needed to convert noradrenaline to adrenaline and will rarely, if ever, secrete adrenaline. The basis of medical treatment is an alpha blocker such as phentolamine or phenoxybenzamine. Beta-blockade by itself could increase the hypertension due to unopposed alpha-activity. The tumour may occur as part of the multiple endocrine adenomata syndrome (MEN-II) in association with hyperparathyroidism and medullary carcinoma of the thyroid. Hypercalcaemia is occasionally found in the absence of hyperparathyroidism or bone secondaries.

57. Hypothermia

A   is defined as a body (core) temperature of 30°C or below
B   causes involuntary shivering of muscles
C   may give rise to delta waves in the ECG
D   is a recognised complication of alcoholism
E   typically produces a systemic alkalosis

58. Prolactin

A   has no established function in males
B   secretion occurs in response to stress
C   in excess can give amenorrhoea
D   is mainly controlled by a hypothalamic releasing hormone
E   secretion may be increased in primary hypothyroidism

59. The following statements regarding diabetes insipidus are correct:

A   the condition is more often produced by hypothalamic than pituitary lesions
B   the treatment of choice in children is chlorpropamide
C   the treatment of choice in adults is DDAVP
D   the absence of nocturia is strong evidence against this diagnosis
E   the symptoms of nephrogenic diabetes insipidus can be improved by thiazide diuretics

60. The following are recognised features of hypothyroidism:

A   menorrhagia
B   ascites
C   cerebellar ataxia
D   clubbing
E   normochromic anaemia

Answers overleaf

57. D

This is generally defined as a core (rectal) temperature less than 35°C. Inability to shiver is one of the causative mechanisms. ECG changes include sinus bradycardia, atrial fibrillation and ventricular fibrillation (particularly below 28°C). The J wave is seen in hypothermic patients as a small positive wave after the R wave; the delta wave is a feature of Wolff-Parkinson-White syndrome. Alcoholism is a common precipitant (remember pancreatitis), as are myocardial infarction, stroke and debilitating infection in the elderly. Hypothyroidism is a rare though important cause. Metabolic acidosis, due in part to tissue hypoxia, is a characteristic finding.

58. A B C E

The release of prolactin from the anterior pituitary is largely controlled by prolactin-inhibitory factor (PIF), probably dopamine, produced in the hypothalamus. When production or release of PIF is deficient, as in hypothalamic or pituitary stalk lesions, hyperprolactinaemia occurs. Prolactin-secreting pituitary microadenomas are also a common cause of hyperprolactinaemia. TRH (thyrotrophin-releasing hormone) releases prolactin and may play a part in the occasional hyperprolactinaemia found in primary myxoedema. The clinical features of hyperprolactinaemia, in addition to amenorrhoea in women, include galactorrhoea, reduced libido and hypogonadism.

59. A C D E

Polyuria throughout the day and night is characteristic in the untreated patient. DDAVP, a synthetic analogue of vasopressin, has an antidiuretic effect for 10 to 12 hours when administered as a nasal spray, and is the treatment of choice. Chlorpropamide potentiates ADH action on the renal tubule, but because of its primary hypoglycaemic action, is best avoided in children. The effect of thiazides is to enhance proximal tubular reabsorption as a result of causing mild salt depletion.

60. A B C E

In addition to normochromic anaemia there is also, in myxoedema, an increased incidence of pernicious anaemia, and menorrhagia may lead to hypochromia. Fluid retention may occur, giving protein-rich pericardial, pleural and peritoneal effusions as well as dependent oedema in the absence of heart failure. An abnormality of lymphatic drainage from interstitial tissues has been implicated.

61. The ocular manifestations of Graves' disease

   A   are nearly always seen when there is pretibial myxoedema
   B   include unilateral exophthalmos
   C   may occur in the absence of hyperthyroidism
   D   are due to thyroid stimulating immunoglobulins
   E   include severe pain in the eye

62. Testicular malfunction

   A   resulting in infertility is usually accompanied by androgen deficiency
   B   resulting in androgen deficiency is usually accompanied by infertility
   C   is the commonest cause of impotence
   D   in Klinefelter's syndrome will show a plasma testosterone response to human chorionic gonadotrophin
   E   occurs in hyperprolactinaemia

63. Characteristic features of heterozygous familial hypercholesterolaemia include

   A   autosomal recessive inheritance
   B   normal ischaemic heart disease risk in affected females
   C   raised plasma LDL concentration at birth
   D   tendon xanthomas in early childhood
   E   defective hepatic LDL receptors

64. The following are recognised features of Wilson's disease:

   A   band keratitis
   B   low urinary copper
   C   liver disease resembling chronic active hepatitis
   D   reduced plasma caeruloplasmin
   E   osteomalacia

Answers overleaf

61. A B C E

Some degree of asymmetry of exophthalmos is a relatively common finding, and occasionally, it may be unilateral, especially at the outset. Loss of vision (malignant exophthalmos) may be due to increasing pressure in the eye causing optic neuritis and atrophy or corneal ulceration and severe pain may be an associated feature. Although there is an increased incidence of high titre thyroid stimulating immunoglobulins (formerly known as LATS) in patients with severe ophthalmic Graves' disease, there is no evidence that these are responsible for the ocular complications.

62. B D E

Infertility is due to failure of the Sertoli cells to produce sperm or to a 'mechanical' disorder, the testosterone-producing Leydig cells often remaining intact. However, an adequate concentration of androgen is necessary for spermatogenesis. Impotence is rarely of endocrine origin or due to testicular disease. The testicular lesion in Klinefelter's syndrome is of the tubules and the interstitial (Leydig) cells may respond to gonadotrophins to produce testosterone (see Q.88).

63. C E

Familial hypercholesterolaemia is an autosomal dominant condition with a gene frequency between 1:300 and 1:500 in the UK. Heterozygotes are affected later and less severely than homozygotes, but ischaemic heart disease risk is increased in all subjects. Tendon and cutaneous xanthomas are rare before the age of ten years in the heterozygote. Screening of neonates (cord blood) allows early detection and treatment when one or both parents are affected. The basic biochemical defect has been localised to the LDL receptor.

64. C D E

The basic abnormality in Wilson's disease is a failure to excrete copper into the bile. Excess copper is toxic and gives rise to various forms of liver disease, a neurological disorder affecting mainly the basal ganglia, Kayser-Fleischer rings in the cornea and renal tubular defects (hence the osteomalacia). The plasma caeruloplasmin and total copper are reduced and the urinary copper excretion is high (see also Q.171).

65. The rate of aldosterone secretion

A   is controlled by the renin-angiotensin system
B   is increased by increased sodium concentrations in the extra-cellular fluid
C   increases when plasma potassium concentrations rise
D   is inversely related to plasma volume
E   is increased by stimulation of the sympathetic supply to the adrenal gland

66. Vasopressin (ADH)

A   is synthesised in the hypothalamus
B   is a steroid
C   increases permeability of the loop of Henle to water
D   is released in response to a fall in blood volume
E   relaxes smooth muscle

67. Hyperuricaemia is a recognised consequence of

A   hypercalcaemia
B   cyanotic heart disease
C   hypoxanthine-guanine-phosphoribosyl transferase (HGPRT) deficiency
D   inhibition of xanthine oxidase
E   glucose-6-phosphatase deficiency (Type I glycogen storage disease)

68. Hypophosphataemic ('vitamin D resistant') rickets is characterised by

A   an autosomal recessive inheritance
B   excessive renal tubular loss of phosphate
C   short stature
D   calcification of inter-spinous ligaments
E   complete resistance to treatment by vitamin D

Answers overleaf

65. A C D

Aldosterone secretion is largely controlled via the renin-angiotensin system, and is inversely related to plasma volume. Plasma potassium concentrations also influence aldosterone release. Aldosterone secretion is greater when the subject is on a low sodium diet. It is the adrenal medulla, not the cortex, which is controlled by the sympathetic nervous system.

66. A D

ADH is a nonapeptide believed to be synthesised in the supraoptic and paraventricular nuclei of the hypothalamus and transported along nerve axons to the posterior hypothalamus. It increases the permeability to water of the renal collecting ducts (both cortical and medullary). The osmolar gradients mean that water leaves the tubule thus concentrating the urine. ADH release stimulated by a fall in blood volume (real or 'apparent') may override osmotic changes inhibiting release, hence the paradox of the hyponatraemia observed in severe volume depletion.

67. A B C E

Hypercalcaemia giving renal failure or due to hyperparathyroidism is associated with hyperuricaemia. Polycythaemia and other myelo- and lymphoproliferative diseases give overproduction of uric acid, and this may also be seen in secondary polycythaemia (which will accompany cyanotic heart disease). Deficiency of HGPRT is the cause of the Lesch-Nyhan syndrome in which gross overproduction of uric acid is associated with choreoathetosis, spasticity, variable mental deficiency and self-mutilation. Children with type I glycogen storage disease (see Q.55) develop gout as a consequence of impaired uric acid excretion secondary to lactic acidosis and ketonaemia, and increased de novo purine synthesis. Xanthine oxidase inhibitors such as allopurinol lower blood urate levels.

68. B C D

Hypophosphataemic rickets is characterised by an X-linked dominant inheritance and affects both males and females. Whereas an excessive tubular loss of phosphate is considered to be the fundamental cause of the condition, it is possible that there is an increased gastro-intestinal loss. Treatment is based on giving large doses of vitamin D together with phosphate supplements, but even with treatment from an early age, it is not thought that normal stature will be obtained. Some cases present in adult life. Calcification of interspinous ligaments occurs, sometimes confused with ankylosing spondylitis or hyperostosis.

69. *Helicobacter pylori*

    A   are found in normals
    B   respond poorly to H_2 antagonists
    C   are found in ectopic gastric tissue in the duodenum
    D   are eliminated by bismuth therapy
    E   cause acute gastritis

70. Concerning pseudomembranous colitis

    A   it is caused by colonisation of mucosa by *Clostridium difficile* bacteria
    B   rectal biopsy is rarely helpful in diagnosis
    C   it requires intravenous vancomycin treatment
    D   it can lead to toxic dilatation of the colon
    E   it is associated with a very low recurrence rate

71. The following are true in liver failure:

    A   a bleeding diathesis is more likely in cirrhosis than after a paracetamol overdose
    B   neomycin is superior to metronidazole
    C   lactulose reduces gut pH
    D   it may be precipitated by constipation
    E   deep coma is associated with opiate analgesia

72. In acute gastroenteritis

    A   patients with an ileostomy are at increased risk from dehydration
    B   refeeding should commence as soon as the appetite returns
    C   oral rehydration therapy (ORT) improves the diarrhoea
    D   antibiotics are contraindicated with Campylobacter infection
    E   commercial ORT is inadequate for children less than 2 years of age

Answers overleaf

69. A C E

Helicobacter pylori are found in 10–30% of normal stomachs on endoscopy. They only colonise gastric tissue and cause an acute gastritis. They are poorly responsive to H_2 antagonists but show some response to bismuth. Eradication is difficult but currently triple therapy with bismuth, metronidazole and amoxycillin is the most effective. They are implicated in ulcer recurrence and possibly in the genesis of peptic ulcers.

70. D

The presence of the bacteria is not sufficient to produce the effects; there must be *Cl. difficile* toxin. Rectal biopsy is often helpful although the condition can be right-sided. Toxic dilatation is an important complication. Treatment is with oral vancomycin or oral metronidazole. The recurrence rate is high.

71. C D E

Liver failure is acute or acute on chronic. Acute liver failure after drugs or viruses is characterised by hypoglycaemia and a generalised bleeding diathesis. Acute on chronic failure demonstrates glucose intolerance and gastrointestinal bleeding related to portal hypertension. Any gut-specific antibiotic is effective; lactulose is useful as it produces a catharsis and an acid caecal pH. The latter reduces the formation of ammonia-dependent bacteria. Opiates are contraindicated and can cause prolonged encephalopathy (see also Q.42).

72. A B

Gastroenteritis in at risk groups (infants, elderly) produces dehydration. ORT, by utilising a glucose-coupled sodium absorption pathway, corrects the dehydration. Commercial preparations are adequate for the treatment of mild/moderate dehydration commonly seen in the UK. Food has little or no effect on the diarrhoea and should be encouraged as soon as practicable. Antibiotics are rarely required but erythromycin is needed for Campylobacter infection with systemic upset.

73. **The following are true of infectious hepatitis:**

    A hepatitis C is food/water borne
    B patients are maximally infectious prior to the onset of jaundice
    C vaccine to hepatitis B may reduce the incidence of hepatoma
    D alkaline phosphatase is rarely more than double the upper limit of the reference range
    E hepatitis D is now the commonest blood borne hepatitis in the UK

74. **Concerning bacterial overgrowth of the gastrointestinal tract**

    A it is rarely seen in the elderly
    B it is more common after partial gastrectomy
    C it does not occur in patients with an ileostomy
    D the most cost-effective investigation is breath hydrogen analysis
    E breath tests cannot easily distinguish bacterial overgrowth from rapid intestinal transit

75. **The following are true statements concerning artificial nutrition:**

    A a low serum albumin indicates malnutrition
    B parenteral nutrition is more effective than enteral nutrition
    C the main complication of TPN is catheter occlusion
    D all enteral feeds are gluten-free
    E the major cause of weight loss in cancer patients is poor nutritional intake

76. **In the investigation of acute gastrointestinal bleeding**

    A a low haemoglobin with a normal MCV indicates recent haemorrhage
    B a raised blood urea indicates proximal bleeding
    C in patients over 60, angiodysplasia of the colon is an important cause
    D angiography is helpful if endoscopy is negative
    E persistent early morning vomiting suggests alcoholic gastritis

Answers overleaf

73. **B C**

Hepatitis C (previously non A-non B) is now the commonest blood borne hepatitis in the UK. Hepatitis D (Delta agent) co-exists with hepatitis B and is rare in the UK. Hepatitis E is food/water borne producing an illness similar to hepatitis A. It is hoped that widespread vaccination against hepatitis B will greatly reduce the incidence of primary hepatoma (see Q.110).

74. **B D E**

A common cause of malabsorption in the elderly is bacterial overgrowth in jejunal diverticula but overgrowth can occur wherever there is decrease in acid production or altered motility. A breath hydrogen analysis after an oral carbohydrate load is cheap and non-invasive.

75. **D E**

A low serum albumin indicates a septic or toxic patient; severe malnutrition, e.g. starvation, does not depress the serum albumin. Enteral nutrition is preferred to parenteral nutrition as it is safer, easier, cheaper and at least as effective. The main complication of TPN is catheter sepsis.

76. **A C E**

An acute upper gastrointestinal bleed leads to a raised urea (increased amino acid absorption and urea generation) and a normochromic normocytic anaemia, but the blood urea will also be raised due to the volume contraction and pre-renal changes accompanying a large bleed from any site. Angiography is rarely helpful if endoscopy is negative; the patient needs to be bleeding at a rate of 0.5 ml/minute in order to be detected on an angiogram.

77. The irritable bowel syndrome

A may follow an episode of infective diarrhoea
B does not affect the stomach
C is a diagnosis which can only be safely made following a normal colonoscopy or barium enema
D is commonly found to have been present in early adult life in patients presenting with diverticular disease in middle age
E rarely presents over the age of 60

78. The following factors influence the rate of gastric emptying of liquids in man:

A the volume of the ingested liquid
B smoking
C the frequency of the migrating motor complex
D the concomitant ingestion of food
E the presence of disaccharides in the liquid

79. The following are true of colonic gas:

A it contains methane in over 90% of subjects
B the hydrogen component is decreased by fasting
C flatus is largely produced by the hydrolysis of complex carbohydrate by brush border enzymes
D production is related to the amount of air swallowed
E production is usually increased in subjects with lactase deficiency

80. In coeliac disease

A there is a biphasic peak of presentation
B gluten withdrawal includes abstinence from oats and maize
C patients well controlled on diet may have a normal jejunal biopsy
D when the diagnosis has been made in infancy, a gluten-free diet can often be withdrawn at puberty
E hyposplenism is a recognised feature

Answers overleaf

77. A

A significant minority of patients relate their symptoms, usually of painless diarrhoea, to an episode of infective diarrhoea often contracted abroad. The whole gut may be involved and gastric symptoms may coexist with colonic ones. A barium enema or colonoscopy is not essential in most patients especially when all the typical features are present in a young person. The diagnosis is common in the elderly but more extensive investigations are required to rule out alternative diagnoses. Despite the similarities between the irritable bowel syndrome and diverticular disease evidence is lacking that the former precedes the latter in individuals.

78. A B D E

Liquid gastric emptying depends on the nature and volume of the liquid, and the presence of tobacco or drugs, e.g. atropine, opiates. Migrating motor complexes clear the fasting gut.

79. B D E

The major factors in the production of intestinal gas are the volume of air swallowed, bacterial colonisation and ingestion of non-absorbable carbohydrates.

80. A C E

A diagnosis of coeliac disease means life long gluten exclusion. Gluten is found in wheat, rye and barley but not in oats, rice and maize. There are two peak ages of presentation: infancy with diarrhoea and growth failure, and 40–60+ years of age where malabsorption or metabolic bone disease may be the major features.

81. In ulcerative colitis

A the rectum is involved in more than 90% of cases
B 5-ASA analogues are more effective at preventing relapses than sulphasalazine
C distal proctitis responds poorly to systemic steroids
D sulphasalazine induces a reversible reduction in sperm count sufficient to cause male infertility
E ileo-anal anastomosis gives equally good results as in Crohn's disease

82. The following are true statements concerning haemochromatosis:

A there is an association with B8 and DW3 HLA antigens
B it is the commonest cause of hepatoma in Britain
C it can lead to pituitary failure
D asymptomatic relatives should be screened for a raised plasma ferritin
E a plasma ferritin value more than five times the upper reference range limit is diagnostic

83. Concerning colonic polyps

A only adenomas have malignant potential
B colonoscopy is the preferred investigation
C polyps larger than 2 cm are more likely to be malignant
D small polyps (less than 2 mm) do not require removal
E red meat and low fibre have been aetiologically linked

84. In chronic pancreatitis

A plasma amylase is often raised even when patients are asymptomatic
B after 50% gland destruction diabetes is inevitable
C histology is important in order to make a diagnosis
D sub-total pancreatectomy provides excellent pain relief at the expense of exocrine insufficiency
E the commonest known aetiological agent in western societies is alcohol

Answers overleaf

81. A C D

Colitis starts in the rectum and may or may not progress proximally. Distal proctitis responds better to local than to systemic drugs. The newer 5-ASA analogues are thought to be as effective as sulpha-salazine at reduced toxicity (see also Q.12 practice exam). Total colectomy with ileo-anal anastomosis is very successful in colitis but may allow severe recurrence of symptoms if used in patients with Crohn's disease.

82. B C D

Haemochromatosis is associated with the A3 and B14 HLA antigens. There is an increase in iron absorption from the gut leading to iron deposition in many organs including the pituitary gland. Serum ferritin is often grossly raised, but as it is an acute phase protein very high concentrations can be seen in many acute conditions. Treatment can reduce complications especially if instituted in the pre-cirrhotic stage.

83. A B C E

The development of most colon cancers from adenomatous polyps is now well established. The larger the polyp the more likely it is to be malignant but even small polyps can grow into large ones! Colonoscopy, because of the ability for polypectomy, is the investigation of choice. Diet, in particular heavy ingestion of red meat and low fibre, is thought to be an important predisposing factor.

84. A E

The commonest known cause of pancreatitis in the UK is alcohol excess. Other known factors include hypercalcaemia and hyper-lipidaemia. In up to 50% of cases no cause is found. Plasma amylase is a very non-specific and insensitive indicator of disease activity. The diagnosis rests on the history, plain X-ray and specific imaging, especially CT scan and ERCP. Histology is difficult to obtain and rarely diagnostic. Over 90% of the gland needs to be destroyed or resected before diabetes ensues (see also Q.22 practice exam).

GENETICS

85. The following are true:

A Gaucher's disease is more common in Ashkenazi Jews
B Erb's muscular dystrophy is X-linked
C ataxia telangiectasia is commoner in men
D defective LDL receptors associated with familial hyper-cholesterolaemia are inherited in an autosomal dominant fashion
E nephrogenic diabetes insipidus is inherited as an autosomal recessive trait

86. The following are more common in men than in women:

A agammaglobulinaemia
B Lesch-Nyhan syndrome
C mixed connective tissue disease
D insulin-dependent diabetes mellitus
E favism

87. The following conditions have an autosomal dominant inheritance:

A familial Mediterranean fever
B neurofibromatosis
C Friedreich's ataxia
D dystrophia myotonica
E haemochromatosis

88. The following are true:

A Klinefelter's syndrome is the result of non-disjunction in either of the parents
B patients with the karyotype 45,XO have an increased risk of coarctation of the aorta
C a Barr body is an inactivated X-chromosome
D patients with the karyotype 47,XYY generally lead normal lives
E the fragile X-syndrome is found predominantly in females

Answers overleaf
43

85. **A D**

Nephrogenic diabetes insipidus is X-linked recessive and familial hypercholesterolaemia, autosomal dominant. Both ataxia telangiectasia and Erb's muscular dystrophy are autosomal recessive conditions (see also Appendix).

86. **A B E**

Agammaglobulinaemia and the Lesch-Nyhan syndrome are X-linked recessive, and therefore more common in males (see Appendix). NB Vitamin D resistant rickets is X-linked dominant. The non-organ specific autoimmune diseases such as mixed connective tissue disease, systemic lupus erythematosus, scleroderma and rheumatoid arthritis are all more common in females. The primary vasculitides, polyarteritis nodosa and Wegener's granulomatosis are commoner in males (4:1). Generally the organ-specific autoimmune diseases (e.g. Graves' disease and Addison's disease) are commoner in women; IDDM affects both sexes equally.

87. **B D**

Familial Mediterranean fever, Friedreich's ataxia and haemochromatosis are autosomal recessive traits. Neurofibromatosis and dystrophia myotonica are inherited as autosomal dominants (see Appendix).

88. **A B C D**

Klinefelter's (47,XXY) may be caused by non-disjunction (failure of the chromosomal pair to separate during meiosis) in either parent. Patients with Klinefelter's are chromatin positive (i.e. have a Barr body visible in the nuclei of their cells). Turner's syndrome is associated with the karyotype 45,XO. The karyotype 47,XYY is associated with tall stature and a below average IQ (1/3) but otherwise patients lead normal lives; a small number of patients with mental retardation have anti-social behaviour. In the fragile X-syndrome there is a characteristic break on one of the Xq arms; the syndrome, which includes mental retardation and macro-orchidism, is found predominantly in males (see also Q.62).

89. *Neisseria gonorrhoeae* **may cause**

   A a pustular rash
   B tenosynovitis
   C meningitis
   D perihepatitis
   E proctitis

90. **Non-gonococcal urethritis may result from**

   A *Mycoplasma hominis*
   B *Mycoplasma genitalium*
   C *Chlamydia trachomatis*
   D *Bifidobacteria*
   E *Ureaplasma urealyticum*

91. **In the diagnosis of syphilis a negative VDRL and a positive TPHA are indicative of**

   A past treated secondary syphilis
   B early primary syphilis
   C untreated tertiary syphilis
   D secondary syphilis
   E infectious mononucleosis

92. **The following organisms cause the following diseases:**

   A *Calymmatobacterium granulomatosis* – lymphogranuloma venereum
   B *Haemophilus ducreyi* – granuloma inguinale
   C *Chlamydia trachomatis* – chancroid
   D *Treponema pallidum* – condylomata acuminata
   E *Pediculosis corporis* – pubic louse (crabs)

Answers overleaf

89. A B C D E

The rash in disseminated gonococcal infection is usually sparse and often associated with tenosynovitis or septic arthritis. Acute perihepatitis (the Fitz-Hugh-Curtis syndrome) may be due to *Chlamydia trachomatis* or *Neisseria gonorrhoeae* and very rarely meningitis and endocarditis may complicate gonococcal infection. Proctitis is a particular complication in homosexuals.

90. B C E

Chlamydia trachomatis accounts for up to half of cases of non-specific urethritis. In the remainder, *Ureaplasma urealyticum* and *Mycoplasma genitalium* are pathogens whereas *Mycoplasma hominis* is not. Bifidobacteria are commensal faecal organisms.

91. A B C

During the primary stage of syphilis all serological tests are initially negative with the exception of the FTA which is then followed by the TPHA and lastly by the VDRL. In the secondary stage of syphilis all serological tests are positive but in tertiary late syphilis, 5–25% of non-specific tests (VDRL) are negative in the absence of past treatment. Following effective treatment the specific tests (TPHA) remain positive whereas the non-specific tests become negative. The non-specific tests (VDRL) may be falsely positive in many infectious diseases whereas the specific tests (TPHA) are not.

92. NONE CORRECT

Calymmatobacterium granulomatosis causes granuloma inguinale, *Haemophilus ducreyi* causes chancroid and *Chlamydia trachomatis* lymphogranuloma venereum. Condylomata lata occur in secondary syphilis and condylomata acuminata are caused by papilloma virus. The pubic louse is *Phthirus pubis* whereas *Pediculosis corporis* is the body louse.

93. **The finding of an intracranial space-occupying lesion in a patient with HIV infection may indicate**

    A *Toxoplasma gondii*
    B *Mycobacterium tuberculosis*
    C *Mycobacterium avium-intracellulare*
    D *Cryptococcus neoformans*
    E Progressive multifocal leuco-encephalopathy

94. **HIV patients are particularly susceptible to the following enteric pathogens:**

    A *Microsporidia*
    B *Isospora belli*
    C *Helicobacter pylori*
    D *Hymenolepsis nana*
    E *Entamoeba hartmanni*

95. **Cryptosporidium**

    A affects the small bowel
    B affects the large bowel
    C has sexual and asexual cycles
    D is an extra-cellular pathogen
    E is susceptible to standard water chlorination

96. **The following would be against the diagnosis of *Pneumocystis carinii* pneumonia in a patient known to be HIV antibody positive:**

    A normal serum lactate dehydrogenase level
    B absence of clinical signs
    C pleural effusion
    D cavities on chest X-ray
    E normal arterial gases after exercise

Answers overleaf

93. A B D E

Toxoplasma gondii tends to cause multiple ring enhancing space-occupying lesions whereas *M. tuberculosis* causes a single enhanced SOL. Lymphoma tends to be non-enhancing and single. *Cryptococcus neoformans* most commonly causes meningitis but can cause multiple enhancing SOLs, and progressive multifocal leuco-encephalopathy, due to JC virus, shows up as non-enhancing low density lesions of the periventricular white matter. A therapeutic trial of antitoxoplasmal therapy (pyrimethamine and sulpha-diazine) is indicated in patients with multiple enhancing SOLs who have positive toxoplasmal serology; response is usually quick. *Cryptococcus* can be diagnosed by looking for the antigen in serum and CSF. Failure to respond to antitoxoplasmal therapy after 2 weeks indicates the need for brain biopsy to elucidate the cause of the lesion (see also Q.38 practice exam).

94. A B

Microsporidia are being increasingly recognised as a cause of protracted small bowel diarrhoea in AIDS patients. The diagnosis has to be made by small bowel biopsy and no established treatment is available. *Isospora belli* should be especially considered in patients from the tropics and is diagnosed by observing the cyst in a stool specimen. Co-trimoxazole treatment is very effective. *H. pylori, H. nana* and *E. hartmanni* may occur in HIV infection but patients are not particularly susceptible nor is the ensuing disease severe.

95. A B C

Cryptosporidium is mainly a small bowel pathogen where it causes prolonged intractable watery diarrhoea, often accompanied by mal-absorption and severe weight loss. Extension of infection to the colon and rectum is relatively common in AIDS and therefore a rectal biopsy is the next step if several stool microscopies are negative for *Cryptosporidium*. Both sexual and asexual cycles take place in the host enabling the organism to be virulent in an immunodeficient host. It is an intracellular pathogen although it lies only just inside the cell. It is extremely resistant to standard chlorination.

96. A C D E

The LDH is invariably raised in *Pneumocystis* pneumonia and the arterial gases abnormal with hypoxaemia after exercise. Cavities are rarely seen in pneumocystis unless the patient has been receiving pentamidine inhalation prophylaxis. The absence of clinical signs is completely compatible with bad pneumocystis and some patients presenting early have a normal chest X-ray. Pleural effusion should suggest another cause, such as *M. tuberculosis* or Kapsosi's sarcoma.

97. **In benign monoclonal gammopathy (monoclonal hypergamma-globulinaemia)**

    A there is a low level of serum albumin
    B there is a marked increase in immature plasma cells in the bone marrow
    C the 'M' band in the serum electrophoretic strip does not show a progressive rise over the course of time
    D there is no anaemia
    E there is no Bence-Jones protein in the urine

98. **The following produce haemolysis in patients with G6PD (glucose 6-phosphate dehydrogenase) deficiency:**

    A primaquine
    B penicillin
    C tetracycline
    D glandular fever
    E nitrofurantoin

99. **In patients with a cold antibody haemolytic anaemia**

    A Raynaud's phenomenon may be a feature
    B a lymphoma is a recognised association
    C IgE antibody is often involved
    D IgG antibodies are sometimes involved
    E recent rubella infection may be relevant

100. **The following are associated with microangiopathic blood changes:**

    A haemolytic-uraemic syndrome
    B severe burns
    C meningococcal septicaemia
    D Down's syndrome
    E typhoid fever

Answers overleaf

97. C D E

In this condition, which may occur in as many as 3% of those over age 70 years, there is an abnormal band of globulin present in the electrophoretic strip. Typically, the level of abnormal globulin (IgG in about 85% of cases) is under 30 g/l and the other serum proteins are normal. This condition is not associated with anaemia, abnormal numbers and types of plasma cells in the marrow, or the presence of Bence-Jones protein in the urine. A percentage have, however, developed multiple myeloma or lymphoma after many years of follow-up (see also Q.230).

98. A D E

Antimalarials were the first group of drugs to be connected with the precipitation of haemolysis in G6PD deficiency. Of the anti-bacterial agents which can safely be given to these patients, penicillin and tetracycline are both useful whilst many sulphon-amide preparations, nitrofurantoin, PAS and chloramphenicol precipitate haemolysis. Many viral infections precipitate haemolysis in G6PD deficiency and glandular fever is a good example of this.

99. A B D E

Raynaud's phenomenon occurs when cold antibodies cause in vivo agglutination at the cold peripheries. These antibodies are usually IgM or IgG in class and the IgM are often associated with lymphoma. The Donath-Landsteiner IgG cold antibody was, in the past, commonly seen with syphilis, but now viral infections such as rubella are the most frequent cause (see Q.230).

100. A B C

Fragmented red cells are seen in the haemolytic-uraemic syndrome and the closely related thrombotic thrombocytopenic purpura. The destruction of small superficial vessels by burns causes breaking up of the red cells as they pass through. In meningococcal sepsis the microangiopathy can be associated with DIC. Micro-angiopathic anaemia occurs in other conditions with DIC such as septic shock, and in malignant hypertension and polyarteritis nodosa.

101. Idiopathic thrombocytopenic purpura (ITP)

A in adults frequently follows a viral infection
B in childhood is characteristically complicated by extensive haemorrhages and a fulminant course
C is characteristically associated with moderate splenomegaly
D is known to occur in children born to a mother previously cured of ITP by splenectomy
E is associated with a reduction of megakaryocytes on bone marrow examination

102. In the investigation of a patient with a bleeding tendency

A a prolonged partial thromboplastin time could indicate haemophilia
B a normal prothrombin time excludes thrombocytopenia
C patients should be asked to refrain from taking aspirin for 14 days
D Hess' test is negative with a coagulation factor deficiency
E a prolonged prothrombin time is a characteristic finding in hereditary haemorrhagic telangiectasia (HHT)

103. In beta-thalassaemia major

A symptoms and signs typically develop at about five years of age
B in children, there is seldom marked enlargement of the spleen
C the mongoloid facies is due to expansion of the facial bones due to marrow hyperplasia
D the serum iron is often raised although the MCH is reduced
E the anaemia is entirely due to decreased haemoglobin synthesis

104. Macrocytosis of red cells is a recognised finding in

A coeliac disease
B ulcerative colitis
C alcoholism
D aplastic anaemia
E patients treated with azidothymidine

Answers overleaf

101. D

Most cases resolve spontaneously in childhood, and the patients usually do not have splenomegaly. Even though the mother may be clinically 'cured' by splenectomy, circulating antibodies may still be present and can affect the baby at the time of delivery. In ITP, megakaryocytes are normal or increased in the marrow.

102. A C D

The partial thromboplastin time is prolonged with deficiencies of the intrinsic system factors including VIII and IX, which do not affect the prothrombin time. The prothrombin time is prolonged with deficiency of the extrinsic system factor VII as well as the common pathway factors X, V and II. Hess' test is abnormal with small vessel abnormality, thrombocytopenia and impaired platelet function. The bleeding disorder in HHT is due to the abnormal mucosal blood vessels. Aspirin causes irreversible inhibition of platelet cyclo-oxygenase and so may cause prolongation of the bleeding time.

103. C D

In severe thalassaemia major, symptoms and signs develop in the first two years of life and marked enlargement of the spleen is very common. Mongoloid facies are typical of all the congenital haemolytic anaemias in which there is marked marrow hyperplasia. Raised serum iron occurs with iron therapy, haemochromatosis, sideroblastic anaemia and the thalassaemias. In beta-thalassaemia major, there is significant under-haemoglobinisation of red cells associated with a very low MCH. The anaemia is due to a combination of ineffective erythropoiesis and haemolysis.

104. A C D E

The macrocytosis of coeliac disease is usually due to folate deficiency. Alcohol makes the red cells large directly, through secondary folate deficiency and with liver disease. In aplasia, younger large red cells are thrown out from the marrow. Azidothymidine may affect red cell morphology via DNA synthesis. A reticulocytosis is also a cause of macrocytosis.

105. Pancytopenia may be caused by

A   folic acid deficiency
B   paroxysmal nocturnal haemoglobinuria (PNH)
C   miliary tuberculosis
D   acute myeloblastic leukaemia
E   haemosiderosis

106. The following are recognised complications of Hodgkin's disease:

A   amyloidosis
B   dermatomyositis
C   cryptococcus infection
D   haemolytic anaemia
E   asthma

107. As compared with chronic myelocytic leukaemia, chronic lymphocytic leukaemia has

A   more marked lymphadenopathy
B   more frequent hypogammaglobulinaemia
C   a more frequent occurrence of a positive Coomb's test
D   more frequent development of a blast crisis
E   a worse prognosis

108. In the differential diagnosis of a raised haematocrit, the following suggest polycythaemia rubra vera:

A   low serum B_{12}
B   high serum iron
C   normal white cell count
D   splenomegaly
E   reduced number of bone marrow megakaryocytes

Answers overleaf

105. A B C D

Important causes of pancytopenia which are potentially reversible also include vitamin B_{12} deficiency, SLE, hypersplenism, and drug-induced marrow aplasia.

106. A C D

There is a T-cell defect in Hodgkin's disease which reflects the long-standing observation of cutaneous anergy in this condition. This probably explains the predisposition to certain infections such as TB, cryptococcosis, toxoplasmosis, pneumocystis, aspergillosis, herpes zoster and disseminated varicella. Treatment undoubtedly aggravates the predisposition. Haemolytic anaemia is much rarer in Hodgkin's disease than with lymphocytic neoplasia.

107. A B C

Patients with chronic lymphocytic leukaemia also tend to be older, the splenomegaly is not as marked, and is painful much less often. Autoimmune thrombocytopenia also can complicate CLL, though less frequently than an autoimmune haemolytic anaemia

108. D

In the classical case, evidence of increased production of all the marrow elements and splenomegaly distinguishes polycythaemia rubra vera from secondary and relative ('stress') polycythaemia. The serum iron tends to be low and the serum B_{12} high due to an increase in the vitamin B_{12} binding proteins.

INFECTIOUS DISEASES & TROPICAL MEDICINE

109. Actinomycosis

   A may be caused by *Actinobacillus actinomycetemcomitans*
   B can be associated with intrauterine devices
   C most commonly affects the lung
   D may be disseminated
   E is best treated with vancomycin

110. The following micro-organisms may cause chronic hepatitis:

   A *Leptospira icterohaemorrhagia*
   B Delta virus
   C Hepatitis B virus
   D Hepatitis C virus
   E Hepatitis E virus

111. The following may result in a lymphocytic meningitis:

   A *Mycobacterium bovis*
   B *Cryptococcus neoformans*
   C *Treponema pertenue*
   D *Brucella melitensis*
   E *Borrelia burgdorferi*

112. The following infections may be contracted from dogs:

   A dysgonic-fermenter 2
   B *Pasteurella multocida*
   C *Echinococcus granulosis*
   D *Leptospira canicola*
   E *Campylobacter foetus*

109. B D
Several species of *Actinomyces* can cause actinomycosis but *Actinobacillus actinomycetemcomitans* is a Gram negative rod that is often found in association with *Actinomyces israelii*; it is not a cause. Pelvic actinomycosis may be associated with IUDs, and can present with anything from a vaginal discharge to a frozen pelvis mimicking malignancy. The disease most commonly affects the cervico-facial area and less commonly the lung or abdomen/pelvis. Disseminated actinomycosis may occur resulting in soft tissue abscesses and optional therapy is benzyl penicillin for prolonged periods. In a penicillin allergic individual, clindamycin is a suitable alternative.

110. B C D
Leptospira icterohaemorrhagia is the commonest leptospira associated with Weil's disease characterised by jaundice and renal failure; chronic hepatitis does not occur. Hepatitis B, C and Delta virus are all spread by blood or contaminated body fluids and they all can result in chronic hepatitis. For acute Delta co-infection (occurring simultaneously with acute hepatitis B) 5% of cases develop chronic hepatitis whereas with Delta super-infection (already hepatitis B surface-antigen carriers) 70% of cases develop chronic hepatitis. 5% of patients with hepatitis B and approximately 30% of those with hepatitis C go on to develop chronic hepatitis. Hepatitis A and hepatitis E do not lead to chronicity (see Q.73).

111. A B D E
Mycobacterium bovis is part of the mycobacterium tuberculosis complex including *M. tuberculosis*, *M. bovis* and *M. africanum*; all can cause clinical and extra-pulmonary tuberculosis. *Treponema pertenue* is the cause of yaws and does not result in neurological disease. Cryptococcal infection is an important cause of a lymphocytic meningitis in immunocompromised persons and those with diabetes mellitus. *Brucellosis* and Lyme disease are other important, but rare, causes of a lymphocytic meningitis.

112. A B C D
Local *Pasteurella* infection of the bite wound complicated by septicaemia, hydatid disease and leptospirosis are all recognised infections that may result from contact with dogs. Dysgonic-fermenter 2 septicaemia is a rare sequelae in patients who have had a splenectomy or are otherwise immunocompromised, and it has a high mortality. Whereas *Campylobacter jejuni* may be contracted from dogs, *Campylobacter foetus* cannot.

113. Botulism

    A is most commonly due to types A, B and E
    B is caused by a spore-forming anaerobic organism
    C is usually associated with fever
    D usually spares the pupillary reactions
    E is invariably fatal

114. The following are true of toxic shock syndrome:

    A a maculo-papular rash is common
    B *Staphylococcus aureus* elaborating enterotoxin C may be isolated
    C hypotension occurs in all patients
    D non-menstrual cases account for one quarter of the total
    E alopecia is common

115. The following rashes may result from *Streptococcus pyogenes* infection:

    A erysipelas
    B erythema marginatum
    C erythema nodosum
    D slapped cheek syndrome
    E ecthyma gangrenosum

116. The following antibiotics are effective against the corresponding organism:

    A teicoplanin – *Escherichia coli*
    B cefuroxime – *Pseudomonas aeruginosa*
    C ciprofloxacin – *Streptococcus pneumoniae*
    D benzyl penicillin – *Streptococcus pyogenes*
    E flucloxacillin – methicillin-resistant *Staphylococcus aureus*

Answers overleaf

113. A B

Spores of *C. botulinum* are ubiquitous in soil and the distribution of types A and B is global. Types A, B and E most commonly produce disease in man; types F and G have only rarely caused human illness. *Clostridium* is a spore-forming anaerobic genus and characteristic features of botulism include the absence of fever, fixed dilated pupils and extreme dryness of the throat due to interruption of cholinergic autonomic transmission. Fatality is approximately 25% if intensive care back up is available.

114. A B C D

Toxic shock syndrome is caused by *S. aureus* producing either TSST-1 or enterotoxins B or C. TSST-1 toxin accounts for all menstrual-related cases and half of the non-menstrual-related cases. Enterotoxins B or C account for the remaining non-menstrual cases. Hypotension is one of the diagnostic criteria which need to be fulfilled, and is present in 100%. Various types of rash can be seen, classically a sunburn-erythema or maculo-papular rash with fine desquamation at day 7–10, especially around the nail-beds. Alopecia does not occur.

115. A B C

Erythema marginatum is one of the major criteria for diagnosing rheumatic fever complicating *S. pyogenes* tonsillitis. Slapped cheek syndrome has been a label given to Parvovirus infection (fifth disease) and *Haemophilus influenzae* Group B cellulitis. Ecthyma gangrenosum is seen in neutropenic patients and results from Gram negative infection, especially *Pseudomonas aeruginosa*.

116. D

Teicoplanin is a cousin of vancomycin and has the same spectrum of action, namely only against Gram-positive organisms. Cefur-oxime is a second generation cephalosporin and as such has no activity against *P. aeruginosa*; ceftazidime, however, does have good activity. Ciprofloxacin has much weaker action against Gram-positives than Gram negatives and is especially weak in its activity against *S. pneumoniae*. Benzyl penicillin is still the treatment of choice for patients with *S. pyogenes* infection. Methicillin-resistant *S. aureus* will be resistant against all beta-lactam antibiotics including fluxloxacillin and the cephalosporins.

117. Life cycles of the following helminths involve the lung:

A *Ascaris lumbricoides*
B *Strongyloides stercoralis*
C *Necator americanus*
D *Ankylostoma braziliensis*
E *Schistosoma japonicum*

118. Rabies

A is invariably fatal
B is caused by a bullet-shaped DNA virus
C may be diagnosed by a corneal smear
D can be passed from person to person
E always causes hydrophobia

119. The following may occur in severe falciparum malaria:

A hypoglycaemia
B hyponatraemia
C haemoglobinuria
D raised intracranial pressure
E liver failure

120. The following organisms not uncommonly cause fever and jaundice:

A *Entamoeba histolytica*
B *Fasciola hepatica*
C *Leptospira icterohaemorrhagia*
D *Clonorchis sinensis*
E *Paragonimus westermani*

Answers overleaf

117. **A B C**

A. lumbricoides, *S. stercoralis* and *N. americanus* all have life cycles that involve spread to the lungs via the bloodstream, breakthrough into the alveoli and then migration to the pharynx to be swallowed again; during this period they mature. *A. braziliensis* is a cause of cutaneous larva migrans and *S. japonicum* a cause of intestinal schistosomiasis.

118. **A C**

The disease is caused by an RNA virus and is invariably fatal. Corneal transplants have been recognised as a method of transmission. Rabies may be either 'furious' or 'dumb' so hydrophobia is not a universal presentation.

119. **A B C D**

Hypoglycaemia complicates malaria in three clinical settings which may overlap: in patients given quinine, in pregnant women and in patients with severe disease, especially young children. Mild hyponatraemia is relatively common and is often accompanied by mildly reduced plasma osmolality. Severe hyponatraemia does occur but is rare; there is no evidence of defective ADH control. Haemoglobinuria (black-water fever) occurs in severe malaria. However, it must be remembered that some patients may be suffering from the oxidant effect of antimalarial drugs when they are G6PD deficient. Raised intracranial pressure is common in cerebral malaria and because of this the justification for doing a lumbar puncture to exclude meningitis has recently been challenged. Hepatic dysfunction is common but clinical signs of liver failure are never seen unless there is concomitant viral hepatitis.

120. **B C D**

Entamoeba histolytica may cause dysentery or an amoebic liver abscess, either of which may result in fever; jaundice, however, is exceptionally rare (see Q.24 and Q.60 practice exam). *Fasciola hepatica* is a sheep liver-fluke whose habitat in animals or man is the biliary system. Cholangitis may occur – as it can with *Clonorchis sinensis* which is a common biliary tract fluke in the Far East. Clonorchis biliary infection may predispose to the development of cholangiocarcinoma. *Leptospira icterohaemorrhagia* is the commonest leptospira causing Weil's disease where renal failure and jaundice are part of the syndrome. *Paragonimus westermani* is the lung fluke.

121. Beta-haemolytic streptococci

A may cause neonatal septicaemia and meningitis
B all possess the Lancefield group A cell-wall antigen
C may have an M-protein in the outer coat which is the main determinant of virulence
D may cause epidermal necrolysis
E are more frequently responsible for glomerulonephritis in the tropics than in temperate climates

122. The following statements about *Escherichia coli* are correct:

A many of the strains are not pathogenic
B it is a non-lactose fermenter
C it characteristically gives rise to foul smelling infections
D it has a recognisable appearance on Gram stain
E it grows anaerobically

123. *Legionella pneumophila*

A has been isolated from the sea and most other types of water
B grows optimally at temperatures of 10–20°C
C can be identified by culture on selective media and by guinea-pig inoculation
D causes Pontiac fever
E is highly infectious and case to case transmission is important during epidemics

124. *Clostridium tetani*

A is pathogenic by virtue of an endotoxin
B is Gram-negative
C bears spores
D is sensitive to tetracycline
E is highly resistant to antiseptics

Answers overleaf

121. A C E

Several strains of streptococci are characterised by their ability to lyse red blood cells; these include organisms with the Lancefield group A antigen (*Str. pyogenes*), group B (*Str. agalactiae*, which can cause serious neonatal infections), and also C and G. Group A streptococci are the most frequently pathogenic in man; the presence of the M-protein in their cellular wall is important for virulence. These organisms may cause skin infections such as erysipelas and impetigo, the latter occurring in epidemic proportions in some tropical countries such that post-infective glomerulonephritis is a frequent complication.

122. E

E. coli belong to the Enterobacteriaceae which include *Salmonella*, *Shigella* and *Proteus* (non lactose-fermenters) and *Klebsiella*, *Enterobacter* and others (lactose-fermenters). All the strains are potential pathogens; foul-smelling pus indicates anaerobes such as *Bacteroides* with which *E. coli* may well be associated. The microscopic appearances are not characteristic and biochemical and serological tests are needed for differentiation from other enterobacteria.

123. C D

Although the natural habitat of *L. pneumophila* is water, moist soil and mud it has not been isolated from sea-water as it is inhibited by sodium chloride; it grows well in warm water but only slowly multiplies where temperatures are below 20°C. Confirmation of the diagnosis in Legionnaire's disease is usually serological, but the organism can be cultured on selective charcoal yeast extract (CYE) media and also after inoculation into guinea pigs. Infection is environmental/nosocomial rather than transmitted from infected patients. Pontiac fever describes a short febrile illness unaccompanied by physical signs or pneumonia and caused by *L. pneumophila*.

124. C D

C. tetani gives clinical effects by means of an exotoxin, tetanospasmin (tetanus toxin). The bacilli are Gram-positive and are spore-bearing; the spores give the bacillus a 'drum-stick' or 'dumb-bell' appearance. The spores are resistant to antiseptics, drying and to a degree, to heat, but the bacilli themselves are not. Although they are sensitive to tetracycline, penicillin is probably the antibiotic of choice.

125. **The following mechanisms are involved in the production of the fluid exudate in acute inflammation:**

   A   increased capillary hydrostatic pressure
   B   increased vascular permeability to protein
   C   breakdown of large molecular tissue proteins
   D   diapedesis
   E   complement activation

126. **The following pathological lesions are characteristic of the following conditions:**

   A   hepatic centrilobular necrosis in Budd-Chiari syndrome
   B   myocardial Aschoff nodules in acute rheumatic fever
   C   neurofibrillary tangles and cerebral amyloid plaques in Alzheimer's disease
   D   centrilobular emphysema in alpha-1 anti-trypsin deficiency
   E   transmural colonic inflammation with histiocytic granulomata in Crohn's disease

127. **The following are characteristic features of malignant tumours:**

   A   abnormal mitoses
   B   anaplasia
   C   reactive hyperplasia in the regional lymph nodes
   D   increased fibrous stroma
   E   invasiveness

128. **In the tuberculous lesion**

   A   initially infiltration with lymphocytes occurs
   B   there is progressive destruction of the organisms by macrophages
   C   caseation consists of dead polymorphs
   D   the presence of numerous giant cells is evidence of healing
   E   the presence of caseation, macrophages and epithelioid cells is diagnostic

Answers overleaf

125. A B C

Diapedesis is the passive movement of red cells out of vessels; complement activation will result in production of chemotactic factors which can induce a directional movement of inflammatory cells. Both occur in acute inflammation, but do not contribute to the fluid exudate.

126. A B C E

Hepatic vein thrombosis is typically responsible for severe centrilobular necrosis. The amyloid plaques characteristic of the cerebral pathology of Alzheimer's disease (see Q.159) may contain prions (proteinaceous infectious agents). Colitis occurring in Crohn's disease is transmural, whereas it is more superficial in ulcerative colitis. Alpha-1 anti-trypsin deficiency is associated with a panacinar form of emphysema.

127. A B E

In malignancy, mitoses tend to be not only abnormal, but numerous. Anaplasia is used to denote lack of resemblance of a malignant tumour to its parent organ. Invasiveness is the hallmark of malignancy. Some malignant tumours produce a marked fibrous reaction (e.g. scirrhous carcinoma of the breast), but this is exceptional.

128. B

There is initial transient acute inflammation with polymorphs. Caseation consists of altered macrophages and dead tissue cells. Fibroblasts, not giant cells, provide evidence of dealing. Although the combination of caseation, macrophages and epithelioid cells is very suggestive of tuberculosis, it is not diagnostic.

129. Renal blood flow

A   is 1/5 to 1/4 of the total cardiac output
B   is distributed evenly to medulla and cortex
C   is increased by sympathetic nervous system overactivity
D   rises with anaemia
E   is constant over the range of blood pressure 90–200 mm Hg

130. Atrial natriuretic factors (ANF)

A   provoke aldosterone secretion
B   inhibit Na/K ATPase in the distal tubular cells
C   may cause renal arteriolar vasoconstriction
D   are undetectable in end-stage renal failure
E   are released from atrial myocytes in concentrations directly proportionate to the atrial pressure

131. In rapidly progressive glomerulonephritis

A   anti-neutrophil cytoplasmic antibodies (ANCA) are often detected
B   there may be evidence of preceding or underlying infection
C   renal prognosis is rarely affected by therapeutic intervention
D   a linear IgM immunofluorescence pattern may be seen on renal biopsy
E   patients often have non-oliguric acute renal failure

132. Incontinence of urine

A   may respond to treatment of a urinary infection
B   is a feature of chronic retention of urine
C   may be induced by a diuretic
D   in the geriatric population, is less common in mobile patients
E   is commonly due to disease of the posterior pituitary

Answers overleaf

129. **A E**
More than 90% of the renal blood flow is directed to the cortex. Stimulation of the renal nerves causes vasoconstriction. In contrast to most tissues, renal blood flow tends to fall with anaemia and rises with polycythaemia thus keeping plasma flow constant. Blood transfusion in chronic renal failure can sometimes lead to a serious fall in renal plasma flow. Autoregulation occurs in the kidney so that the blood flow remains constant over the range of blood pressures 90–200 mm Hg.

130. **NONE CORRECT**
Atrial natriuretic peptides are released from myocytes in response to atrial stretch rather than absolute atrial pressure. They have a variety of actions within the kidney including vasorelaxation of renal arterioles, modulatory effects upon GFR, and they diminish the ADH-induced water reabsorption in the collecting ducts. Natriuretic effects are seen in the distal tubule (inhibition of aldosterone-mediated Na reabsorption) but there is no action on the Loop of Henle. Massive ANF activity is observed in patients with congestive cardiac or end-stage renal failure.

131. **A B**
The characteristic histology of extensive glomerular epithelial cell proliferation (hence 'crescentic glomerulonephritis') may be associated with infection (SBE, post-streptococcal disease) and occurs in other acute systemic disorders such as SLE and Henoch-Schönlein purpura. ANCA may be present in vasculitides (microscopic polyarteritis, Wegener's granulomatosis) and anti-GBM antibodies seen in Goodpasture's syndrome are IgG. Patients usually develop oligo-anuria and early treatment with immunosuppressive drugs with or without plasma exchange may considerably influence outcome.

132. **A B C D**
Inflammatory changes in the bladder mucosa due to infection, catheters, stones etc. may give urgency incontinence. In a patient whose control of micturition is tenuous, the use of diuretics will often precipitate incontinence. Any obstruction to bladder outflow such as chronic prostatic enlargement may lead to chronic retention and overflow incontinence. Diabetes insipidus must be incredibly rare as a cause of incontinence. Far more important are the above, and gynaecological stress incontinence, with faecal impaction often playing a role in the elderly.

133. In classical (distal type 1) renal tubular acidosis (RTA) in adults, the following are characteristic findings:

    A polyuria
    B aminoaciduria
    C hyperchloraemia
    D uraemia
    E ureteric colic

134. The following statements about Goodpasture's syndrome are correct:

    A pulmonary haemorrhage occurs in less than half the patients
    B the serum complement level is generally normal
    C renal transplantation is contraindicated
    D plasma exchange is effective in controlling nephritis but not lung haemorrhage
    E intercurrent infection may lead to disease relapse

135. The following factors in a patient with acute renal failure would favour the use of peritoneal dialysis (PD) rather than haemodialysis:

    A myocardial infarction
    B chronic bronchitis
    C advanced age
    D hypotension
    E hypercatabolic renal failure

136. The following are typical associations of polycystic disease of the kidneys in adults:

    A subarachnoid haemorrhage
    B nephrolithiasis
    C polycythaemia
    D liver failure
    E nephrotic syndrome

Answers overleaf

133. A C E

Aminoaciduria is found as an associated proximal tubular defect in proximal (type II) RTA. In distal RTA there is failure of hydrogen-ion excretion; this abnormality can be primary, or far ·more commonly occurs as a result of conditions which predominantly affect the renal medulla and interstitium, such as chronic reflux uropathy, hypercalcaemia, hypokalaemia, obstructive uropathy, Sjögren's syndrome and other interstitial nephritides. Considering the primary form, the polyuria is due to impaired osmotic concentrating ability, in part due to hypokalaemia, which also gives muscle weakness. Nephrocalcinosis and urinary stones form due to hypercalciuria, alkaline urine and a low urinary citrate excretion. They may contribute to glomerular failure in some cases, but uraemia is not a typical early feature. The other major problems arise from osteomalacia.

134. B E

Two-thirds of patients with anti-GBM disease have pulmonary haemorrhage and plasma exchange in addition to immunosuppressive therapy may be required for life-saving control. Transplantation is an effective treatment for end-stage renal failure where anti-GBM titres are low; in patients where titres are elevated intercurrent infection frequently triggers clinical relapse.

135. A C D

Haemodialysis is more haemodynamically stressful to patients than PD and should be avoided, generally, when the circulatory state is at particular risk, after a myocardial infarct, in the elderly and in the hypotensive. PD, splinting the diaphragms, can lead to respiratory problems even with 1 litre exchanges. It may also not provide adequate urea clearance to correct the uraemia if urea production is especially high. The optimal urea clearance with PD is about 25–30 ml/min compared with 100 ml/min or more for haemodialysis.

136. A B C

Berry aneurysms and urinary stones occur in about 10% of cases. Although liver cysts are found in perhaps a third of cases, they rarely give rise to symptoms and probably never to liver failure. This is in contrast to the much rarer polycystic disease of childhood, where liver failure and portal hypertension due to hepatic fibrosis may be the dominant clinical features.

137. **The following are recognised associations of patients with calcium containing urinary stones:**

    A   a positive family history
    B   a persistently low urinary pH
    C   hyperuricosuria
    D   small bowel malabsorption
    E   medullary-sponge kidney

138. **Ureteric obstruction is a characteristic complication of**

    A   gastrojejunostomy
    B   analgesic nephropathy
    C   schistosomiasis
    D   renal transplantation
    E   aortic aneurysm

139. **The following are true of the nephrotic syndrome:**

    A   a better prognosis in children
    B   an association with chronic liver disease
    C   it is rare in tropical countries
    D   remission of proteinuria may occur with cyclosporin A
    E   there may be an accompanying hypercoagulable state

140. **In a patient found to be severely uraemic, the following would indicate chronic renal disease:**

    A   pericarditis
    B   hyperphosphataemia
    C   skin pigmentation
    D   urinary osmolality 300 mosmol/kg
    E   radiological osteodystrophy

Answers overleaf

137. A C D E
There is a marked tendency for idiopathic hypercalciuria, which is a predominantly male disease and the commonest single cause of calcium stones, to run in families. Persistently acid urine is a feature of uric acid stone formers. Calcium phosphate tends to precipitate in alkaline urine whereas calcium oxalate stones do not depend on urine pH. Factors that predispose to oxalate stones include hyperuricosuria either dietary or due to gout, and increased absorption of oxalate from the bowel in malabsorption states (see also Q.133 and Q.138).

138. A B C D E
Intestinal by-pass operations may result in secondary hyper-oxaluria with formation of calcium oxalate stones. Ureteric obstruction occurs in analgesic nephropathy due to sloughed papillae. In schistosomiasis (due to *S. haematobium*), fibrosis occurs in the bladder and ureters, stones are common, and in Egypt, carcinoma of the bladder develops. Ureteric necrosis, due to disturbance of the vascular supply, is a not uncommon complication of transplantation. Leakage from an abdominal aortic aneurysm may be important in the pathogenesis of some cases of retroperitoneal fibrosis (see also Q.17).

139. A B D E
The commonest lesion in children is minimal-change nephropathy which responds well to corticosteroids; cyclosporin A has been used successfully to treat relapses in adults. Chronic hepatitis B surface antigenaemia may cause a membranous glomerulonephritis, and this lesion can also result from *Plasmodium malariae* infection (Quartan nephropathy) which is the most frequent cause of nephrotic syndrome worldwide. Levels of clotting factors are increased and fibrinolytic components reduced in nephrotic states, and as the intravascular fluid volume is also contracted thrombosis is a frequent complication (e.g. renal vein thrombosis).

140. C E
It can sometimes be difficult to distinguish acute renal failure and an acute presentation of end-stage renal disease, although a full history often provides the necessary clues. Other evidence of longstanding renal failure includes the presence of renal osteo-dystrophy, neuropathy, anaemia and small kidneys. Pericarditis may occur in both acute and chronic renal failure.

141. Concerning acute renal failure

A   serum complement levels are usually low
B   acute renal inflammatory disease (glomerular or interstitial) is the commonest cause
C   mortality is low if dialysis is instituted early
D   it may result from paracetamol poisoning
E   renal recovery is rarely expected

142. The following are important factors in determining the suitability of a patient for renal transplantation:

A   hepatitis B surface antigen positive status
B   previous membranous glomerulonephritis
C   high titres of lymphocytotoxic antibodies in the patient
D   full matching at HLA-A locus between patient and potential donor
E   evidence of peripheral vascular disease

143. In the radiological investigation of patients with renal disease the following are true statements:

A   IVU is the most useful first-line investigation in both acute and chronic renal failure
B   DMSA will demonstrate cortical scarring in reflux nephropathy
C   ultrasound, DTPA and MAG3 scanning may all demonstrate urinary tract obstruction
D   IVU may be more useful than ultrasound in the investigation of haematuria
E   serial isotope scanning may be more reliable than IVU in the detection of renal artery stenosis

144. An increase in the ratio of plasma urea to creatinine is found in patients

A   on corticosteroid therapy
B   with severe liver disease
C   with intestinal haemorrhage
D   with uretero-colic anastomosis
E   with extensive burns

Answers overleaf

141. D

Acute renal failure is most commonly the result of circulatory stress such as hypovolaemic, cardiogenic or septic shock (acute tubular necrosis). If the patients are adequately supported renal function usually returns, but as many are severely ill with multi-organ failure overall mortality remains high. Paracetamol can directly cause tubular necrosis.

142. C E

If lymphocytotoxic antibodies directed against HLA antigens are present in the recipient's serum then the chances of a successful transplant may be reduced; immuno-absorption has been used to remove the antibodies in selected cases. The most important loci for the purposes of donor/recipient matching are HLA-B and HLA-DR. Mesangiocapillary glomerulonephritis can re-occur in a renal transplant (as can focal segmental sclerosis, IgA nephropathy, Goodpasture's and the vasculitides, although in the latter examples a rise in auto-antibody titre will herald disease recurrence) but as in the case of previous hepatitis B infection this should not preclude transplantation. Marked aortic and iliac vessel atheroma may render the patient untransplantable.

143. B C D E

In advanced chronic renal failure injected contrast may not be concentrated by the kidneys; IVU may also exacerbate renal damage in some forms of acute renal failure. DMSA is avidly taken-up and bound by renal tissue and provides accurate evidence of structure. DTPA and MAG3 are rapidly concentrated and excreted by the kidneys and so allow assessment of differential blood flow and function (including the excretory phase). IVU provides information from the whole of the urinary tract in the search for urothelial malignancy in patients with haematuria.

144. A C D E

In addition to glomerular filtration, the major determinant of plasma creatinine concentration is the rate of production which depends on skeletal muscle mass. Urea production, however, rapidly rises in catabolic states (with injury, heart failure, infection and corticosteroid therapy) and with increased gastrointestinal absorption of nitrogen (GI haemorrhage, uretero-colic anastomosis, and high protein diet). Urea production falls in severe liver disease. Urea excretion falls in dehydration due to increased renal tubular re-absorption, hence increasing the plasma urea/creatinine ratio.

145. **A low level of serum complement (C₃) is a characteristic finding in**

    A minimal change glomerulonephritis
    B mesangio-capillary (membrano-proliferative) glomerulonephritis
    C sub-acute infective endocarditis
    D interstitial nephritis
    E microscopic polyarteritis

146. **The following are recognised associations of some hypokalaemic states:**

    A juxta-glomerular hypertrophy
    B vacuolation of glomerular epithelial cells
    C acidosis in fulminant colitis
    D hypotension
    E hypovolaemia

147. **Serum osmolality might be considerably greater than the osmolarity in the following conditions:**

    A renal failure
    B ethanolic intoxication
    C severe nephrotic syndrome
    D monoclonal gammopathy
    E diabetic ketoacidosis

148. **With metabolic acidosis a normal anion-gap may suggest**

    A renal tubular acidosis
    B treatment with acetazolamide
    C diarrhoea
    D salicylate poisoning
    E uraemia

Answers overleaf

145. B C

A low serum complement level is seen in disorders in which there is complement fixation and deposition within glomeruli. This pattern occurs in glomerulonephritis associated with SLE, infected ventriculo-atrial shunts and in post-streptococcal disease. One variety of mesangio-capillary glomerulonephritis is characterised by the presence of a protein in the serum (C_3 nephritic factor) that can induce C_3 cleavage in vitro.

146. A C D E

Pathological changes occurring in severe hypokalaemia are predominantly in the tubular cells and interstitium. Alkalosis is usually present in those cases of hypokalaemia not due to intrinsic renal disease (Conn's and Cushing's syndromes, pyloric stenosis, diuretic or exogenous steroid excess), but acidosis is observed with severe diarrhoea because of excessive bicarbonate loss. In Bartter's syndrome there is considerable salt wasting, and untreated cases are hypotensive due to hypovolaemia; renin secretion is over-stimulated with consequent hypertrophy of the juxtaglomerular apparatus.

147. B C D

The osmolality is a direct measure of the osmolar concentration of 1 kg of plasma whereas the osmolarity is an estimation derived from the measured Na, K, urea and glucose concentrations. The osmolarity will thus be unreliable in conditions where pseudohyponatraemia is present, such as that due to hyperlipidaemia (which will occur in severe nephrotic syndrome) or hyperproteinaemia. The osmolality will also take account of plasma constituents that are not normally present (e.g. alcohol).

148. A B C

The anion-gap is calculated by subtracting the measured plasma anionic concentration (bicarbonate and chloride) from the added serum sodium and potassium value, and should be in the range 10–16 mmol/l. In the presence of metabolic acidosis a normal or low anion gap would indicate hyperchloraemic acidosis (such as with diarrhoea or renal tubular acidosis), whereas an enlarged gap would signify the presence in plasma of a normally undetected anion/acid that might be contributing to the acidosis (e.g. lactic, salicylic or ketoacids, unmeasured uraemic toxins). Acetazolamide inhibits bicarbonate reabsorption in the renal tubule.

149. A lesion of the right half of the seventh cervical segment of the spinal cord may

A impair position sense in the right leg
B cause a positive Hoffman's sign on the right
C abolish the right abdominal reflexes
D impair temperature sensation below the level of the lesion on the right
E cause clonus at the right ankle

150. Characteristic features of occlusion of the left middle cerebral artery in a right-handed individual include

A a hemiplegia that affects the leg more than the arm
B paralysis of conjugate gaze towards the left
C anosagnosia
D acalculia
E alexia

151. Chorea is a recognised complication of

A prochlorperazine
B metoclopramide
C amitriptyline
D selegeline
E tetrabenazine

152. The following are recognised presentations of a non-secreting pituitary adenoma:

A CSF rhinorrhoea
B binasal visual field defect
C anorexia
D petit mal epilepsy
E sudden monocular blindness

Answers overleaf

149. A B C E

A right sided cord lesion will produce ipsilateral pyramidal and dorsal column signs and contralateral spinothalamic signs – the Brown-Sequard syndrome. Hoffman's sign indicates a pyramidal lesion above the eighth cervical segment.

150. D E

The motor and sensory abnormalities affect predominantly the face and arm. The cortical representation for the leg is parasaggital and is supplied by the anterior cerebral artery. Both the motor area for speech in the frontal lobe and the language areas in the temporal and parietal lobes are affected producing a global aphasia, including difficulties with reading and calculation. Conjugate gaze to the opposite side of the lesion is affected. Anosagnosia describes the loss of ability to recognise or to acknowledge bodily defect and is a non-dominant parietal lobe disorder.

151. A B C D

Chorea may be caused by drugs which increase striatal dopamine activity (L-dopa, selegeline, tricyclic antidepressants) or stimulate striatal dopamine receptors (bromocriptine). Tardive chorea is caused by dopamine blocking agents (including the commonly used metoclopramide and prochlorperazine) and is thought to be caused by receptor hypersensitivity. Tetrabenazine is used in the treatment of Huntingdon's chorea.

152. A B C E

A pituitary tumour may erode into the sphenoid sinus and cause CSF rhinorrhoea. Although temporal visual field defects are the most common, any visual field defect may be caused by chiasmal compression and distortion. Anorexia may be caused by hypothalamic involvement and monocular blindness by pressure on the ophthalmic artery (see also Q.20. practice exam).

153. Pseudobulbar palsy

    A is caused by bilateral lesions of the corticospinal tracts
    B may cause nasal speech
    C causes an absent gag reflex
    D may be caused by multiple sclerosis
    E may cause fibrillation of the tongue

154. Diabetic amyotrophy

    A causes predominantly distal weakness and wasting
    B is associated with raised CSF protein levels
    C has a poor prognosis for recovery
    D causes loss of the ankle jerks
    E causes impotence

155. Absent ankle jerks are associated with extensor plantar responses in

    A tabes dorsalis
    B vitamin B_{12} deficiency
    C motor neurone disease
    D lesions of the conus medullaris
    E ataxia telangiectasia

156. There is a known association between chronic alcoholism and

    A painful myopathy
    B auditory hallucinosis
    C cerebellar degeneration
    D downbeating nystagmus
    E hypoglycaemia

Answers overleaf

153. B D

Pseudobulbar palsy is caused by bilateral lesions of the cortico-bulbar tracts. Typical causes are small vessel cerebral vascular disease, multiple sclerosis and cerebral trauma. Examination reveals upper motor neurone signs affecting the bulbar structures. Nasal speech is caused by palatal weakness and may be found in both bulbar and pseudobulbar palsy.

154. B

Diabetic amyotrophy is thought to be caused by occlusion of the vasa nervorum of the proximal lumbar plexus and/or the femoral nerve, causing infarction. Pain in the thigh followed by weakness and wasting of the quadriceps and loss of the knee jerk are typical clinical features. Recovery over a period of months is the rule. The CSF protein is raised in two thirds of patients with diabetes mellitus but does not correlate with the presence or the severity of neuropathy.

155. B D

Deficiency of vitamin B_{12} causes degeneration of large fibre sensory neurones in the peripheral nerves and their central connections in the dorsal columns of the spinal cord, causing loss of tendon jerks and sensory ataxia. With more prolonged deficiency the pyramidal tracts degenerate causing an extensor plantar response. At the conus medullaris, the spinal root entry zones and the pyramidal tracts are in close proximity and may be damaged by a small lesion such as a neurofibroma. Taboparesis and Friedreich's ataxia are other causes of an extensor plantar response and absent ankle jerks.

156. A B C E

Alcohol abuse is a well recognised cause of an acute painful myopathy. Auditory hallucinations are a prominent feature of delerium tremens. Hypoglycaemia is believed to result from the blockage of gluconeogenesis when there are depleted liver glycogen stores (see Q.55). Children are particularly prone to alcohol-induced hypoglycaemia. Downbeating nystagmus is a sign of a lesion at the foramen magnum.

157. **Unilateral ptosis is a recognised finding in**

   A   syringobulbia
   B   cluster headache
   C   Bell's palsy
   D   cavernous sinus thrombosis
   E   thoracic outlet syndrome

158. **In aneurysmal subarachnoid haemorrhage**

   A   multiple aneurysms are detected in about 20% of patients
   B   vertebrobasilar circulation aneurysms are detected in about 30% of patients
   C   dementia is a late complication
   D   stroke may be precipitated by angiography
   E   ST segment elevation may be present on the electrocardiograph

159. **In Alzheimer's disease**

   A   social misconduct and personality change are typical features
   B   the plantar response is typically extensor
   C   myoclonus is common in the late stages
   D   neurofibrillary tangles are diagnostic
   E   temporo-parietal hypometabolism on positron emission tomography is a typical finding

160. **The median nerve**

   A   supplies the muscles of the hypothenar eminence
   B   supplies adductor pollicis
   C   typically supplies the 1st and 2nd lumbricals
   D   lies deep to the extensor retinaculum at the wrist
   E   supplies the 1st and 2nd palmar interossei

Answers overleaf

157. A B D E

Causes of a Horner's syndrome include damage to the sympathetic pathways in the medulla, such as in syringobulbia, lesions of the first thoracic root in the thoracic outlet syndrome, and external carotid artery dilatation in cluster headache. The IIIrd nerve runs in the lateral wall of the cavernous sinus and may be damaged in cavernous sinus thrombosis.

158. A C D E

Over 90% of aneurysms lie on the anterior part of the circle of Willis and multiple aneurysms are detected in 20% of patients. Vasospasm is common between the fourth and tenth days post haemorrhage and may be worsened by angiography and surgery, causing stroke. ST segment elevation on ECG is thought to be due to sympathetic hyperactivity caused by intracranial haemorrhage, however, the most characteristic changes are deep symmetrical inverted T waves. Normal pressure hydrocephalus due to arachnoid granulation blockage causing dementia, gait disturbance and incontinence is a late complication.

159. C E

Alzheimer's disease causes an early degeneration of the limbic system and temporo-parietal neocortex. Decreased brain activity in these areas appears to predate degeneration and may be detected by positron or single photon emission tomography. In the late stages patients develop extrapyramidal features (rigidity, hypokinesia and stooped posture) and myoclonus. The cortico-spinal tracts are not affected. Neurofibrillary tangles are also found in other degenerative diseases including progressive supra-nuclear palsy and dementia pugalistica. Features of frontal lobe dysfunction suggest an alternative diagnosis such as lobar atrophy or Pick's disease.

160. C

The median nerve enters the palm by passing underneath the flexor retinaculum and supplies the muscles of the thenar eminence and the 1st and 2nd lumbricals. The muscles of the hypothenar eminence, the interossei, the adductor pollicis and the 3rd and 4th lumbricals are supplied by the ulnar nerve, which enters the palm superficial to the flexor retinaculum.

161. **In myasthenia gravis**

    A most patients will become symptom free following thymectomy
    B anti-acetylcholine receptor antibodies are detected in about 50% of patients
    C anti-smooth muscle antibody is associated with an increased risk of thymoma
    D there is damage to the nicotinic acetylcholine receptors
    E increased weakness may follow the introduction of treatment with corticosteroids

162. **Lewy body dementia**

    A is a rare cause of dementia in patients over 70 years
    B may present with typical idiopathic Parkinson's disease
    C may present with cognitive change without extrapyramidal features
    D is rarely associated with hallucinosis
    E is typically associated with fluctuating cognitive impairment

163. **Causes of periodic (repetitive) complexes on the EEG include**

    A Pick's disease
    B hepatic coma
    C Creutzfeldt-Jakob disease
    D subacute sclerosing panencephalitis (SSPE)
    E progressive multifocal leukoencephalopathy (PML)

164. **The following treatments may reduce the severity of relapse in multiple sclerosis (MS):**

    A pulsed high dose methylprednisolone
    B adrenocortical trophic hormone (ACTH)
    C hyperbaric oxygen
    D azathioprine
    E linoleic acid supplementation

Answers overleaf

161. D E

Myasthenia gravis is associated with anti-nicotinic acetylcholine receptor antibodies in around 90% of patients. Anti-striated muscle antibodies suggest the presence of thymoma. Around 30% of patients are rendered symptom free by thymectomy – mostly those with thymic hyperplasia. Corticosteroids cause decreased acetylcholine release from the presynaptic terminal which may cause a temporary worsening of weakness before the immuno-suppresive actions take effect.

162. B C E

Lewy body dementia may cause up to 25% of dementia in patients over 70 years and is associated with Lewy bodies (an inclusion body typically detected in the brains of patients with Parkinson's disease) throughout the cerebral cortex as well as in the substantia nigra. Patients may present with typical idiopathic Parkinson's disease or with cognitive change alone. Hallucinations and a fluctuating mental state are characteristic clinical features. Lewy bodies have been more easily recognised in recent years because of the development of staining for ubiquitin, a degradation protein found within all inclusion bodies.

163. B C D

Periodic complexes are typically detected in Creutzfeldt-Jakob disease, SSPE, herpes simplex encephalitis and hepatic coma. In the latter the complexes often have a triphasic appearance. In Pick's disease the EEG is invariably normal whereas in PML the recording shows a diffuse slowing of rhythms.

164. E

The only treatment proven to reduce the severity of relapse in MS is dietary supplementation with linoleic acid. Recent trials have shown both azathioprine and hyperbaric oxygen to be ineffective and potentially dangerous. Corticosteroids and ACTH bring forward remission following relapse but do not modify the overall course of the disease.

165. Following surgery for an abdominal aortic aneurysm, a 63 year old man developed weakness of the legs. Likely signs on examination two weeks later include

A the presence of a urinary catheter
B impaired temperature sensation in the legs
C fasciculation of the quadriceps
D weakness of hip extension greater than hip flexion
E impaired position sense at the great toe

166. A 16 year old girl presents with jerks of the arms on waking and three generalised tonic-clonic seizures. The treatment of choice is

A carbamazepine
B phenytoin
C sodium valproate
D clonazepam
E any of the above

167. Recognised associations of an eighth nerve schwannoma include

A a similar lesion on the contralateral side
B Lisch nodules (iris hamatomatas)
C meningiomas
D phaeochromocytomas
E ash-leaf spots

168. The following statements are true in internuclear ophthalmoplegia (INO):

A there is often nystagmus greatest in the abducting eye
B adduction is slow or restricted
C bilateral INO is diagnostic of multiple sclerosis (MS)
D INO may be a feature of myasthenia gravis
E INO is associated with retraction nystagmus

Answers overleaf

165. A B

The artery of Adamkewicz, the major abdominal tributary of the anterior spinal artery, is occasionally damaged by aortic aneurysms and their repair. The anterior spinal cord at the lower thoracic level is typically infarcted, producing pyramidal and spinothalamic signs below the level of the lesion and sphincter dysfunction. Prognosis for recovery is poor.

166. C

Juvenile myoclonic epilepsy typically presents around puberty with myoclonic jerks and generalised tonic-clonic seizures on waking. The interictal EEG shows polyspike wave complexes and photo-sensitivity is common. There is a family history of seizures in about a quarter of patients. The treatment of choice is sodium valproate on which about half of patients will become seizure free.

167. A C

There are at least two genetically distinct forms of neuro-fibromatosis (NF). Patients with NF-2 are at risk of bilateral eighth nerve schwannomas and other brain tumours, including meningiomas. Cutaneous manifestations are rare. Patients with NF-1 have prominent cutaneous manifestations including cafe-au-lait macules, neurofibromas, axillary freckles and Lisch nodules but brain tumours, apart from optic pathway gliomas, are rare. Phaeochromocytomas occur in NF-1. Ash-leaf spots are hypo-pigmented macules which occur in tuberous sclerosis.

168. A B D

INO is caused by a lesion in the medial longitudinal bundle, which prevents messages from the pontine centre for lateral gaze reaching the contralateral medial rectus part of the IIIrd nerve nucleus. Messages reach the ipsilateral VIth nerve nucleus normally. Hence, with a lesion of the left medial longitudinal bundle, causing a left INO, there will, on right lateral gaze, be normal abduction of the right eye but slow or restricted adduction of the left eye. Ataxic nystagmus, greatest in the abducting eye is often an associated feature. Bilateral INO is typical but not diagnostic of MS and may be detected in myasthenia gravis. Retraction nystagmus is a sign of a lesion in the dorsal midbrain.

OPHTHALMOLOGY

169. **Primary open-angle (simple) glaucoma**

    A characteristically gives rise to signs before symptoms
    B is a familial disorder
    C may present as an acute painful red eye
    D gives characteristic visual field defects
    E is usually treated initially by surgery

170. **Anterior uveitis is the most characteristic ocular manifestation of**

    A rheumatoid arthritis
    B sarcoidosis
    C systemic lupus erythematosus
    D Behcet's disease
    E ankylosing spondylitis

171. **Abnormalities of the optic lens are recognised in**

    A homocystinuria
    B hypoparathyroidism
    C dystrophia myotonica
    D hepato-lenticular degeneration (Wilson's disease)
    E congenital rubella

172. **The following would characteristically result in visual field defects:**

    A craniopharyngioma
    B retrobulbar neuritis
    C tertiary syphilis
    D Gaucher's disease
    E Weber's syndrome

Answers overleaf

169. A B D

By far the commonest variety of primary glaucoma, this disease is one of insidious onset and progression. There are arcuate scotomata, peripheral field loss, and excavated pale optic discs. Central vision is preserved until late, which tends to delay presentation. Treatment is essentially medical and based on parasympathomimetic and beta blocker eyedrops. Carbonic anhydrase inhibitor drugs are also used.

170. B D E

Keratoconjunctivitis sicca is common and episcleritis and scleritis are important manifestations of rheumatoid disease. In sarcoidosis the eye is involved in 10–25% of cases, the usual lesion being acute or chronic uveitis; occasionally choroido-retinitis, sicca syndrome and optic nerve lesions are seen. Although SLE can produce inflammatory changes anywhere in the eye, the most frequent sign of ocular involvement is retinal exudates (cytoid bodies). Recurrent anterior uveitis is the most commonly disabling complication of Behcet's disease.

171. A B C D E

Downward dislocation of the lens is characteristic of homocystinuria and cataracts may form at a later stage. Cataracts can develop as a result of chronic hypocalcaemia, which is also associated with papilloedema, and are also the main optic manifestation of myotonic dystrophy. Maternal rubella infection in the first trimester of pregnancy may result in a host of congenital abnormalities including cataracts. Kayser-Fleicher rings are the corneal copper deposits characteristic of Wilson's disease but 'sun flower' cataracts that do not disable vision are also recognised in this condition (see Q.64).

172. A B

Bitemporal hemianopia can result from optic chiasmal compression by a craniopharyngioma. Retrobulbar neuritis, which most frequently accompanies multiple sclerosis, can lead to central scotoma which may also result from optic atrophy, optic nerve compression and choroido-retinitis. Posterior uveitis may also occur rarely in tertiary syphilis but the characteristic ocular abnormality is the Argyll-Robertson pupil. Weber's syndrome refers to infarction of one half of the midbrain, resulting in ipsilateral oculomotor nerve palsy, contralateral hemiplegia and paralysis of upward gaze. Conjunctival pingueculae may be associated with Gaucher's disease.

173. Delayed bone age (skeletal maturity) is found in the following conditions:

A growth hormone deficiency
B precocious puberty
C hypothyroidism
D metatarsus varus
E familial short stature

174. Pertussis immunisation is contraindicated in a child

A with atopic eczema
B who develops fever of 40°C within 36 hours of 1st dose of the triple vaccine
C whose maternal uncle is an epileptic
D who develops a severe local reaction at the site where the 1st dose of the triple vaccine was administered
E who had hypocalcaemic fits in the neonatal period

175. In cystic fibrosis

A the sweat chloride concentration is characteristically elevated
B rectal prolapse may be a presenting feature
C it may present with bile stained vomiting in the neonatal period
D the affected males are usually infertile
E the gene is located on chromosome number 5

176. Strawberry naevi (cavernous haemangiomata)

A have a significant predisposition to malignant change
B often enlarge during the first year of life
C should be treated by surgical excision
D are associated with mental retardation
E if very large, may be associated with thrombocytopenia

Answers overleaf

173. **A C**

Bone age or skeletal maturity is estimated by comparing the appearance of bones on an X-ray of the left hand and wrist with those in a standard atlas, or by the more accurate bone-scoring method of Tanner and Whitehouse. Delay in bone age is found in children with growth hormone deficiency and hypothyroidism. Bone age is usually normal in familial or genetic short stature, and advanced in precocious puberty.

174. **B D**

Absolute contraindications to pertussis immunisation are:
  (i) Severe general reactions. Fever equal to or more than 39.5°C within 48 hours of vaccine; anaphylaxis; generalised collapse; prolonged unresponsiveness; prolonged inconsolable screaming and convulsions occurring within 72 hours.
 (ii) Severe local reaction to the preceding dose. An area of extensive redness and swelling which becomes indurated and involves most of the antero-lateral area of the thigh or the major part of the circumference of the upper arm.
(iii) Unstable neurological condition. Unlike symptomatic hypoglycaemic fits, the outcome of hypocalcaemic fits in the neonatal period is usually good i.e. not associated with neurodevelopmental problems.

175. **A B C D**

Sweat sodium and chloride concentrations are characteristically elevated. Rectal prolapse is a recognised clinical feature of cystic fibrosis in infancy. Approximately 10% of cases present in the neonatal period with intestinal obstruction due to meconium ileus. Aspermia is a uniform finding in males, resulting from obliteration of the vas deferens. The gene is located on chromosome number 7 (see also Q. 215).

176. **B E**

Strawberry naevi may be single or multiple. The lesions usually enlarge during the first year and usually resolve spontaneously over the next few years. Surgical treatment is not recommended unless the lesion involves vital structures e.g. the larynx. There is no predisposition to malignant change. Large or rapidly expanding naevi can lead to platelet consumption and depletion of circulating clotting factors (Kasabach-Merritt syndrome).

177. Idiopathic infantile hypercalcaemia (William's syndrome)

A   is attributed to increased renal calcium reabsorption
B   has an association with patent ductus arteriosus
C   the affected infant may have distinctive facial features
D   hypercalcaemia may be treated with a low calcium and vitamin D diet
E   is often associated with raised plasma cholesterol concentration

178. Causes of fits in the neonatal period include

A   hypomagnesaemia
B   Werdnig-Hoffman disease
C   maternal heroin addiction
D   necrotising enterocolitis
E   excessive use of cows' milk products

179. Systemic onset juvenile rheumatoid arthritis (Still's disease) is typically associated with

A   salmon-pink macular rash
B   splenomegaly
C   positive antinuclear factor
D   high intermittent fever
E   rheumatoid nodules

180. Causes of cataracts in childhood include

A   congenital rubella infection
B   *Chlamydia trachomatis*
C   galactosaemia
D   Down's syndrome
E   cystinosis

Answers overleaf

177. C D E

Hypercalcaemia in idiopathic infantile hypercalcaemia (IH) is caused by increased gastrointestinal calcium absorption. Urinary calcium excretion in IH is usually increased and can lead to nephrocalcinosis. The hypercalcaemia is treated with a calcium and vitamin D deficient diet, until it resolves, usually in the first few years of life. Patients with William's syndrome have 'elfin-like' facial features, mental retardation and aortic stenosis. Not all the patients with William's syndrome are hypercalcaemic. The reason for elevated plasma cholesterol concentrations in some infants with IH/William's syndrome is not known.

178. A C E

Hypomagnesaemia leads to decreased parathyroid hormone (PTH) production and end-organ resistance to the action of PTH, which in turn leads to hypocalcaemic fits. High phosphate concentration in cows' milk leads to hypocalcaemia. Symptoms of narcotic withdrawal in the neonate include irritability, yawning, sweating, fever, diarrhoea, vomiting and fits. Werdnig-Hoffman disease is a degeneration of the anterior horn cells and cranial motor nuclei.

179. A B D

Clinical features of systemic onset juvenile rheumatoid arthritis include high intermittent fever and salmon-pink macular rash in >90%. Other features include lymphadenopathy, splenomegaly, pericarditis, myocarditis, pleuritis, and anaemia. Antinuclear and rheumatoid factor tests are usually negative. Rheumatoid nodules are usually absent.

180. A C D

Congenital rubella infection, galactosaemia and Down's syndrome are all recognised causes of cataracts in childhood. *Chlamydia trachomatis* infection acquired in utero or during passage through the birth canal can cause neonatal conjunctivitis (ophthalmia neonatorum). In cystinosis, crystals of cystine are deposited in the cornea, conjunctiva, sclera and retina (see also Q.171).

181. Congestive heart failure in infancy

A   is commonly associated with peripheral pitting oedema
B   causes hepatomegaly
C   is always associated with central cyanosis
D   is a recognised complication of hypoplastic left heart syndrome
E   often presents with tachypnoea

182. Manifestations of symptomatic HIV infection in childhood include

A   hepatosplenomegaly
B   failure to thrive
C   persistent oral thrush infections
D   lymphocytic interstitial pneumonia
E   developmental delay

183. The human parvovirus (B 19)

A   is the causative agent for roseola infantum
B   causes a desquamative rash
C   is known to cause aplastic crisis in children with haemolytic disease
D   is known to cause polyarthralgia in children
E   is known to cause the haemolytic-uraemic syndrome (HUS) in 15% of the affected children

184. Concerning gastro-oesophageal reflux in infancy

A   it is a recognised cause of failure to thrive
B   the majority of the infants require surgical treatment
C   haematemesis may be a presenting feature
D   it is characteristically associated with para-oesophageal hiatus hernia
E   it is a recognised cause of recurrent pneumonias

Answers overleaf

181. B D E

Tachypnoea and hepatomegaly are cardinal features of heart failure in infancy. Peripheral pitting oedema is less common in infants than in older children and adults. Infants with hypoplastic left heart syndrome develop heart failure because of poor left ventricular function.

182. A B C D E

The symptoms of HIV infection in children are often non-specific and include persistent diarrhoea, repeated upper respiratory infections, persistent fever, hepatosplenomegaly, lymphadeno-pathy, oral thrush and failure to thrive. As in adults, opportunistic bacterial, viral, protozoal and fungal infections are a common problem. Developmental delay, loss of developmental milestones and spastic paraparesis may either be due to direct invasion of the brain by the HIV virus or to opportunistic CNS infections e.g. cerebral toxoplasmosis.

183. C D

Roseola infantum or the 'sixth disease' is caused by the human herpes virus 6. The human parvovirus (B 19) causes erythema infectiosum or the 'fifth disease' which is characterised by a mild febrile illness, erythematous rash on the cheeks (slapped cheek appearance) and a fine reticular rash over the extremities. It is also known to cause aplastic crisis in haemolytic disease, and poly-arthralgia. The epidemic form of HUS is thought to be caused by verotoxin-producing *E.coli*.

184. A C E

Failure to thrive, oesophagitis, haematemesis and recurrent aspir-ation pneumonias are all recognised complications of gastro-oesophageal reflux. It is usually associated with a sliding hiatus hernia. Indications for surgical treatment (fundoplication) include failure of intensive medical treatment, oesophageal stricture and chronic aspiration pneumonias.

185. In Down's syndrome

A there is an increased incidence of hypothyroidism compared with normal subjects
B there is an increased risk of atlanto-axial instability
C hypertonia is a characteristic feature in the newborn
D ileal atresia is the commonest gastrointestinal malformation
E survival to adulthood is complicated by premature senility

186. Features of hyaline membrane disease of the newborn include

A chest wall recession
B decreased lung compliance
C increased lung surfactant
D hyperpyrexia
E liability to chest infections in later childhood

187. At the age of eight months, a baby can be expected to

A roll over from front to back
B pick up a small bead between thumb and finger
C sit up with a straight back
D say up to five words clearly
E feed itself with a spoon

188. In congenital adrenal hyperplasia

A a male infant appears normal at birth
B testicular hypertrophy occurs
C a female infant typically has clitoral hypertrophy and fusion of labia minora
D the presentation may be with saline depletion and shock in the early weeks of life
E ACTH is effective treatment

Answers overleaf

185. A B E

Primary hypothyroidism and the incidence of other autoimmune disorders is increased. Atlanto-axial instability occurs in 10–20%. Hypotonia is one of the most constant signs in Down's syndrome babies. Duodenal atresia is the commonest gastrointestinal malformation. Premature senility and degenerative brain changes similar to Alzheimer's disease occur in older patients.

186. A B

Lung compliance, i.e. the ability of the lung to expand and collapse in response to pressure changes is markedly reduced in hyaline membrane disease, and this is associated with decreased lung surfactant. The temperature is often subnormal. After recovery the lungs are normal in structure and function, and there is no increase in susceptibility to infections later.

187. A C

Rolling over (the denotative righting reaction) is acquired by most babies at five months of age, but the ability to pick up a bead between finger and thumb usually only at about one year. Babies sit up unsupported at eight months and usually feed themselves with a spoon after one year. Most babies say their first words clearly around 12–14 months, but five words will often not be clearly spoken until 14–16 months.

188. A C D

Male infants with this condition may show slight penile enlargement and pigmentation, but both are very easily overlooked and passed as normal. The testicles are normal in size and will slowly atrophy if the condition is untreated due to the circulating androgens. The salt-losing syndrome occurs in about 50% of infants with the 21-hydroxylase block variety. ACTH is, of course, ineffective in treatment (and harmful) since the primary defect is of an enzyme required to elaborate cortisol. It is necessary, therefore, to give cortisol in some form to these patients.

189. Typical features of dementia include

A   selective impairment of recall
B   perseveration of themes
C   generalised cortical atrophy
D   disorientation in place
E   depression

190. The following statements regarding compensation neurosis are correct:

A   it has a recognised association with major rather than minor accidents
B   it occurs particularly after head injuries sustained at work
C   settlement of a compensation claim is followed by improvement in patients with severe symptoms
D   malingering accounts for at least 30% of cases
E   irritability is a recognised feature

191. Grief reaction

A   is typically self-limiting
B   characteristically includes denial
C   is best treated with tricyclic antidepressants
D   typically includes suicidal ideas
E   is a form of psychosis

192. Typical features of alcohol withdrawal include

A   dehydration
B   visual hallucinations
C   passivity feelings
D   tremor
E   confabulation

Answers overleaf

189. A B C D E

In dementia, there is a selective impairment of memory for recent events in the early stages. Later, this generalises and eventually extends to loss of memory for distant events too. There is difficulty in adapting to new situations, so the patient persists or perseverates with old themes. The memory loss is accompanied by disorientation, which may be in time, place, or person. Depression is quite common in early dementia. The dementing process is a result of slowly progressive cortical disease resulting in cortical atrophy.

190. B E

The incidence of compensation neurosis has an inverse relationship with the severity of the injury. It is twice as common after industrial injuries as after road traffic accidents. Little recovery is found in patients with severe symptoms even after settlement of the compensation claim. The main symptoms are headaches, dizziness, poor concentration and irritability. Malingering is not a common occurrence, and the mechanisms involved in producing these symptoms are subconscious ones.

191. A B D

The initial stage of a grief reaction is a period of numbness with little or no emotional reaction. This is the period of denial. Subsequent stages follow to a state of depression, and suicidal ideas are often expressed. These may reflect feelings of guilt or identification with the dead person. The reaction is self-limiting although there may be delays up to several years. The treatment of choice would be some form of psychotherapy or counselling. The reaction is neurotic rather than psychotic.

192. A B D

Delirium tremens on withdrawal from alcohol includes a coarse, persistent tremor of the hands. Often, the patient experiences visual hallucinations such as seeing animals crawling on the floor or the bedclothes. There is free perspiration, oliguria and dehydration. Passivity feelings are features of schizophrenia. Confabulation, part of Korsakoff's syndrome, is a result of chronic alcohol abuse, not of acute withdrawal (see also Q.156).

193. Good prognostic signs in schizophrenia include

A   early onset
B   depressive features
C   echolalia
D   preservation of affect
E   visual hallucinations

194. The following information may reasonably be given to patients starting a course of tricyclic antidepressants:

A   they should expect the drug to take effect within 24 hours
B   they should avoid cheese
C   they may experience a dry mouth at first
D   their skin may become sensitive to sunlight
E   it may help them to lose weight

195. Factors indicating an increased risk of suicide in a depressed patient include

A   a direct statement of intent to commit suicide
B   hopelessness
C   pressure of serious physical illness
D   living alone
E   presence of paranoid delusions

196. Agoraphobia

A   usually starts before puberty
B   occurs more often in women than men
C   can be effectively treated by systematic desensitisation
D   becomes worse during periods of depression
E   can usually be traced back to traumatic events in childhood

Answers overleaf

193. B D

The patient with early onset schizophrenia usually suffers more chronic personality deterioration. The presence of affective change, depression or mania seems to indicate preservation of personality and a better prognosis. There is no evidence that any individual symptom such as visual, rather than auditory, hallucinations influences prognosis. Echolalia is usually a symptom of organic brain damage (see Q.46 practice exam).

194. C

Tricyclic anti-depressants take at least ten days to have their effect. They have no interaction with food as do the monoamineoxidase inhibitors, and do not induce sensitivity to sunlight as do the phenothiazines. They have no direct effect on weight, except that as the depression resolves, the appetite should improve. Initial side effects include dry mouth, but this usually clears up after a few days. Patients should be given this information so that they are encouraged to persist with treatment.

195. A B C D

The most obvious warning sign of suicide is a direct statement of intent by the patient. There is no truth in the theory that people who talk about killing themselves actually do not do it. The presence of a feeling of hopelessness is a predictor of both immediate and subsequent suicide. Of the social factors, positive family history of suicide, prolonged physical illness and living alone indicate a higher risk. Paranoid delusions can occur in depressive illness, but do not have any special significance in assessing suicide risk.

196. B C D

Agoraphobia generally commences suddenly in adult life following a recent traumatic event. There is a large preponderance of women patients, and a worsening of symptoms can occur as a result of other emotional changes such as a period of depression. Treatment is very difficult, but the condition can respond to desensitisation by systematically introducing the patient to the feared situation.

197. The following are characteristic features of hypomania:

A flight of ideas
B thought insertion
C sexual promiscuity
D delusions of bodily illness
E sleep disturbance

198. Puerperal psychosis

A usually begins within two weeks after childbirth
B is commonly accompanied by clouding of consciousness
C has a favourable prognosis
D characteristically includes auditory hallucinations
E characteristically includes obsessional ruminations

199. Anorexia nervosa

A occurs exclusively in females
B tends to be accompanied by episodes of over-eating
C is characterised by apathy and lassitude
D may lead to hypokalaemia
E is a cause of primary amenorrhoea

200. Korsakoff's syndrome is

A a recognised complication of alcoholism
B due to vitamin B_{12} deficiency
C characterised by generalised deterioration of intellect
D characterised by recent memory defect
E associated with nystagmus

Answers overleaf

197. A C E

Flight of ideas, where there is an excessively fluent flow of thoughts and ideas, but with some thread of connection between them, is characteristic of hypomania. Thought insertion is a first rank symptom of schizophrenia. Overactivity and a sense of grandiosity can lead to sexually promiscuous behaviour. Delusions of bodily illness are a feature of depression, not mania. The manic patient is so active he tends to have very little sleep and can become ill through exhaustion.

198. A B C D

The majority of puerperal psychoses begin within the first two weeks after childbirth, and rarely in the first two days. The illness usually starts with a period of delirium. The outlook is favourable. Auditory hallucinations are frequently experienced, but obsessional ruminations are not part of the clinical picture.

199. B D E

The anorectic patient is typically alert and active in spite of severe emaciation. There may be episodes of hyperactivity. Nonetheless, there is a high incidence of depression and, terminally, weakness and apathy predominate. Hypokalaemia is commonly found, often due to self-induced vomiting or purgation. Amenorrhoea, primary and secondary, is a characteristic feature, and may occur before significant weight loss. The typical endocrine findings are low FSH, LH and oestrogen levels; evidence suggests that the fault lies in hypothalamic control of the anterior pituitary.

200. A D E

Korsakoff's syndrome is characterised by a severe memory defect both retrograde and antegrade, i.e. an inability to retain new information. Other mental functions may be more or less intact. Confabulation is common, but not invariable. With Korsakoff's syndrome in chronic alcoholism, beri-beri and prolonged vomiting, Wernicke's encephalopathy is frequently associated giving nystagmus, ocular palsies and ataxia (see also Q.192). Vitamin B_1 (Thiamine) deficiency is the major aetiological factor. Korsakoff's syndrome also occurs after head injuries and cerebral anoxia and with cerebral tumours.

201. The following are recognised associations:

A   small left pneumothorax and audible systolic 'click'
B   acute pancreatitis and adult respiratory distress syndrome
C   sarcoidosis and bronchial obstruction
D   Dressler's (post-myocardial infarction) syndrome and pleural effusion
E   nitrofurantoin and chronic pulmonary fibrosis

202. Cavitating lung lesions are characteristic of

A   systemic lupus erythematosus
B   squamous cell carcinoma
C   Wegener's granulomatosis
D   progressive massive fibrosis
E   'shock lung'

203. The following are recognised treatments of choice:

A   lung lavage in alveolar proteinosis
B   oral corticosteroids in symptomatic bronchopulmonary aspergillosis
C   nebulised pentamidine in severe pneumocystis pneumonia (PCP)
D   ampicillin in psittacosis
E   methylprednisolone in sepsis induced ARDS

204. Surgical resection of carcinoma of the bronchus is contraindicated in the presence of the following:

A   SVC obstruction
B   hoarseness with immobile left vocal cord
C   mediastinal nodes >1.5 cm in diameter on CT scan
D   hypercalcaemia
E   raised mobile right hemi-diaphragm

Answers overleaf

101

201. A B C D E

'Crunching sounds' or 'systolic clicks' can be heard synchronously with the cardiac cycle at the apex with a small left pneumothorax (with or without mediastinal emphysema). Enzymes released in acute pancreatitis damage, amongst other tissues, the lung surfactant and capillaries. Bronchial obstruction in sarcoidosis can be due to endobronchial disease or external compression by enlarged lymph nodes. Dressler's syndrome has amongst its other features, fever, pericarditis, pneumonitis and arthralgia. Pulmonary fibrosis is a recognised complication of chronic nitrofurantoin therapy. An acute lung reaction can occur within hours of taking the drug; there are chest X-ray changes and often a blood eosinophilia.

202. B C D

Other causes of cavitating lung lesions include tuberculosis, staphylococcal and Klebsiella pneumonia, fungal infections such as aspergillosis, septic and non-septic pulmonary infarction, rheumatoid nodules, and progressive massive fibrosis in silicosis and coalminers' pneumoconiosis.

203. A B

Lung lavage is the single most useful therapy in alveolar proteinosis. Symptomatic bronchopulmonary aspergillosis requires steroids in the therapy regimen. Parenteral pentamidine or cotrimoxazole should be given in PCP if the PaO_2 is less than 8.0 kPa (60 mm Hg). Tetracycline is the treatment of choice in psittacosis. Several recent studies have confirmed the lack of benefit with methylprednisolone in ARDS due to sepsis.

204. A B

Resection is contraindicated if mediastinal nodes are involved, signs of which are pressure on the SVC or recurrent laryngeal nerve. CT cannot confirm malignant involvement by size alone. Hypercalcaemia may be due to tumour PTH production rather than metastatic bone deposits. Unlike phrenic nerve palsy, the raised hemi-diaphragm of a collapsed lung caused by proximal tumour compression is mobile, and does not contraindicate resection.

205. **The following statements about hypertrophic osteoarthropathy are correct:**

A   oat cell carcinoma of the bronchus is the commonest cause
B   the arthropathy is typically symmetrical
C   the joint pain is relieved by vagotomy below the origin of the recurrent laryngeal nerve
D   gynaecomastia is a recognised association
E   pretibial myxoedema is a recognised association

206. **Haemoptysis is a characteristic of**

A   byssinosis
B   idiopathic pulmonary haemosiderosis
C   aspergilloma
D   Goodpasture's syndrome
E   asbestosis

207. **The following are typical features of cryptogenic fibrosing alveolitis (diffuse idiopathic interstitial fibrosis):**

A   recurrent haemoptysis
B   stridor
C   finger clubbing
D   'honeycomb' lungs radiologically
E   circulating rheumatoid factor

208. **Recognised occupational causes of asthma include**

A   isocyanates
B   platinum salts
C   soldering flux
D   asbestos
E   beryllium

Answers overleaf

205. B C D

Hypertrophic osteoarthropathy is characterised by clubbing, gynaecomastia, sub-periosteal new bone formation and symmetrical arthropathy, the pain of the latter being helped by vagotomy below the origin of the recurrent laryngeal nerve. Squamous cell carcinoma of the bronchus is the commonest cause. It should be distinguished from 'thyroid acropachy' of which pretibial myxoedema forms a part.

206. B C D

Haemoptysis is an important part of the clinical picture of idiopathic pulmonary haemosiderosis, aspergilloma and Goodpasture's syndrome (pulmonary haemorrhage and glomerulonephritis with anti-basement membrane antibody (see Q.134). It would be atypical in byssinosis, which is due to inhalation of dusts of cotton, flax or hemp, or in asbestosis, unless complicated by lung cancer.

207. C D E

The characteristic symptoms and signs are dyspnoea, cyanosis, clubbing and basal crepitations. Honeycombing is a non-specific x-ray appearance of many diffuse lung diseases in an advanced stage. Rheumatoid factor is found in an appreciable percentage of cases; frank rheumatoid arthritis sometimes is associated. There is also an association with chronic active hepatitis, Hashimoto's disease and renal tubular acidosis.

208. A B C

Isocyanates are used in polyurethane foam manufacture and platinum in the electronics and chemical industries. An increasing number of organic dusts are being recognised as causes of occupational asthma. Asbestosis gives diffuse lung fibrosis and berylliosis is a granulomatous disease resembling sarcoidosis.

209. In alpha₁-antitrypsin deficiency

A   emphysema is usually most marked in the lower lobes
B   the mode of inheritance is autosomal recessive
C   the onset of pulmonary symptoms typically occurs in childhood
D   atopy is a characteristic association
E   smoking plays a synergistic role in the development of emphysema

210. Characteristic features of pulmonary hypertension include

A   dominant S wave in ECG lead V_1
B   large 'a' wave in jugular venous pulse
C   exertional dyspnoea
D   angina
E   clubbing

211. Pleural calcification occurs in

A   silicosis
B   asbestosis
C   haemothorax
D   tuberculosis
E   haemosiderosis

212. Transfer factor

A   increases throughout childhood
B   is higher in males than females
C   is reduced by exercise
D   is a precise measure of the diffusion characteristics of the alveolar membrane
E   is transiently elevated in idiopathic pulmonary haemosiderosis (IPH)

Answers overleaf

209. A E

Alpha$_1$-antitrypsin deficiency is associated with severe panacinar emphysema and is an autosomal co-dominant condition with incomplete penetrance. Patients present in early adult life, usually before the age of 40, and the emphysema is more severe in cigarette smokers. Children with alpha$_1$-antitrypsin deficiency are prone to severe liver disease such as neonatal hepatitis and cirrhosis.

210. B C D

The ECG changes might include right axis deviation, dominant R waves over the right sided precordial leads and evidence of right atrial hypertrophy. Exertional dyspnoea in pulmonary hypertension without lung or left sided heart disease, has been attributed to ischaemia of the muscles of respiration. Finger clubbing is likely if the cause of the pulmonary hypertension is destructive lung disease or cyanotic heart disease, but is not a sign of pulmonary hypertension itself.

211. B C D

Silicosis causes calcification of intra-thoracic lymph glands producing an 'egg-shell' appearance. The extensive pleural plaques of asbestosis with interlobar, diaphragmatic and pericardial location is often diagnostic. Haemosiderosis gives intra-pulmonary calcification.

212. A B E

Transfer factor (TLCO) is a measure of gas exchange which substitutes carbon dioxide for oxygen and depends on alveolar ventilation (oxygen to lungs), blood flow (oxygen to body), Hb (oxygen carriage) and lung volume (surface area for gas exchange). Matching of ventilation and blood flow is much more important than the membrane diffusion characteristics. Its elevation in IPH is due to uptake by Hb in the alveoli.

213. The following statements are true:

A   the vagus nerve is responsible for normal bronchial tone
B   there are 18 bronchopulmonary segments
C   most of the alveoli in the adult lung are present at birth
D   the surface markings of the right middle lobe approximate to the axilla
E   the major component of surfactant is dipalmitoyl lecithin

214. In the acquired immunodeficiency syndrome

A   the lung is affected at some stage in the illness in over two thirds of cases
B   pneumocystis pneumonia (PCP) is an acute onset, rapidly progressive illness
C   atypical mycobacterial infection is usually due to *M. xenopii* or *M. kansasii*
D   broncho-alveolar lavage (BAL) plus transbronchial biopsy (TBB) are diagnostic in up to 90% of cases with pneumocystis pneumonia
E   *mycobacterium tuberculosis* typically occurs at an earlier stage than pneumocystis pneumonia

215. In heart-lung transplantation (HLT) for cystic fibrosis

A   pleurectomy is a recognised contraindication
B   the recipient's heart is not usually suitable for re-transplant-ation
C   azathioprine is included in maintenance immuno-suppression
D   obliterative bronchiolitis is a major long term complication
E   the ion transport defect responsible for cystic fibrosis typically develops in the transplanted lungs within 18 months

216. In asthma

A   mortality has been falling steadily over the past ten years
B   the new long-acting inhaled bronchodilators are recom-mended for first line therapy
C   bacterial infections are a common cause of acute attacks
D   more than 90% of patients have hyperreactive airways
E   salbutamol and terbutaline act on adrenergic nerve endings to relax airway smooth muscle

Answers overleaf

213. A B E

The cholinergic activity of the vagus nerve maintains normal bronchial tone. There are five lobes, divided into 18 bronchopulmonary segments (10 right, 8 left). At birth there are some 25 million alveoli which increase in the adult to 300 million per lung. The right middle lobe extends from the 5th rib in the axilla to the 4th costochondral junction superiorly (horizontal fissure), and to the 6th costochondral junction inferiorly (oblique fissure). Surfactant is a mixture of phospholipids, with dipalmitoyl lecithin predominating.

214. A D E

The lung is affected in more than 70% of AIDS patients. The symptoms of pneumocystis pneumonia (dyspnoea, dry cough and fever) usually develop insidiously over several weeks. Nontuberculous mycobacterial infection is found in 10–20% of AIDS patients during life, the commonest being *M. avium-intracellulare*. The combined diagnostic yield of BAL and TBB in PCP is greater than 90%. Tuberculosis occurs earlier in the natural history of HIV infection than PCP, with a better preserved CD4 count (see also Q.96).

215. A C D

Both pleurectomy and pleurodesis are contraindications to HLT at present. Retransplantation of the recipient's heart is a standard procedure (the 'domino operation'). Azathioprine and cyclosporin form routine maintenance immunosuppressive therapy. As for HLT in general, obliterative bronchiolitis is a major long term problem. The increased potential difference across the respiratory mucosa, typical of cystic fibrosis, has remained normal in transplanted lungs up to 2 years after the procedure (see also Q. 175).

216. D

Asthma mortality has not improved significantly over the past 50 years. Long-acting inhaled bronchodilators are currently only recommended when inhaled steroids have provided inadequate control. Viral infections commonly precipitate attacks. Virtually all symptomatic asthmatics have hyperreactive airways, as do a significant number of the normal population. There is no direct adrenergic innervation of the airways by beta-2 agonists acting on adrenergic receptors.

217. The following may be manifestations of rheumatoid arthritis:

A erythema multiforme
B erythema nodosum
C episcleritis
D digital gangrene
E amyloidosis

218. Radiological bone erosions are a typical finding in

A hyperparathyroidism
B Wegener's granulomatosis
C gout
D systemic lupus erythematosus
E psoriatic arthritis

219. Carpal tunnel syndrome is

A often bilateral in amyloidosis
B a cause of wasting of abductor pollicis brevis
C diagnosed by finding delayed ulnar nerve conduction
D a possible cause of pain in the forearm
E associated with diabetes

220. The following are features of systemic sclerosis:

A calcinosis
B an association with intra-abdominal malignancy
C myopathy
D central nervous system involvement
E an association with primary biliary cirrhosis

Answers overleaf

217. C D E

Episcleritis is a benign, relatively common manifestation of rheumatoid arthritis. Scleritis is rarer and more serious, being a manifestation of vasculitis, as is digital gangrene. Amyloidosis is a complication of many chronic inflammatory conditions (see also Q.47 practice exam).

218. A C E

Gout and psoriatic arthritis can both cause relatively coarse erosion of bone adjacent to affected joints. A finer bony destruction, especially subperiosteal, is typical of the osteitis fibrosis cystica of hyperparathyroidism. Important sites to examine are the middle phalanges, the symphysis pubis and skull. Erosions have been reported in SLE but are rare and are not typical. Wegener's granulomatosis is typified by necrotising lesions of nasal mucosa, lung, kidney, joints, skin and nervous system.

219. A B D

The common causes of carpal tunnel syndrome are pregnancy, hypothyroidism, acromegaly and rheumatoid arthritis. Diabetes is associated with problems in the hand – cheiroarthropathy, not of carpal tunnel syndrome. Delayed median nerve conduction is the hallmark and abductor pollicis brevis wasting largely contributes to the thenar eminence wasting. It is difficult to explain how the pain often radiates as proximally as the elbow, but it is a common symptom.

220. A C E

The CREST syndrome (Calcinosis, Raynaud's, Oesophageal involvement, Sclerodactyly, Telangiectasia) is generally a benign disorder not associated with the systemic involvement seen in scleroderma. Whereas the feature of myopathy runs throughout the spectrum of connective tissue diseases, CNS complications are not a feature of systemic sclerosis and are more characteristic of SLE. However, systemic sclerosis can cause resistant malignant hypertension which could, in turn, cause cerebrovascular disease. Polymyositis and dermatomyositis in adults are associated with underlying malignancy.

221. Mixed connective tissue disease

A commonly presents with Raynaud's phenomenon
B is diagnosed by the presence of anti-ribonucleoprotein antibodies
C typically has raised titres of anti-DNA antibodies
D carries a better prognosis than systemic sclerosis
E typically causes renal impairment

222. Drug-induced systemic lupus erythematosus is

A equally common in men and women
B significantly more common in fast than slow acetylators
C not generally complicated by renal disease
D caused by sulphonamides
E irreversible, even after drug withdrawal

223. Joint pain is a recognised feature of

A idiopathic thrombocytopenic purpura
B Christmas disease (factor IX deficiency)
C acute post-streptococcal glomerulonephritis
D sarcoidosis
E amyloidosis

224. The following statements regarding pseudo-gout (chondrocalcinosis) are correct:

A acute arthritis involves the knee more often than other joints
B hydroxyapatite crystals are found in the synovial fluid
C the disease may mimic osteoarthritis of the hands
D there is a recognised association with primary hyperparathyroidism
E colchicine provides effective prophylaxis against acute attacks

Answers overleaf

221. A B D

Mixed connective tissue disease is a clinical syndrome with Raynaud's, myositis and swollen digits as common abnormalities. It is typified by the presence of antibodies to ribonucleoprotein. Some cases progress to systemic sclerosis. Renal involvement is uncommon.

222. A C D

Drug-induced SLE is equally common in men and women whereas 'idiopathic' SLE has a 9:1 female to male preponderance. The list of drugs that may precipitate lupus includes sulphonamides, isoniazid, griseofulvin, hydralazine, penicillamine procainamide and carbamazepine. Slow acetylators are more prone and slower metabolism of the drugs is important. Drug-induced SLE is virtually never complicated by renal disease. Withdrawal of the offending drug leads to disappearance of the disease, but complete reversal has been recorded as taking up to 2 years in some cases of hydralazine-induced SLE.

223. B D E

Christmas disease is indistinguishable clinically from haemophilia, and haemarthrosis is a major clinical problem. Arthritis is not a feature of thrombocytopenia, although prominent in Henoch-Schönlein purpura. Arthralgia and arthritis occur in sarcoidosis with erythema nodosum and, more chronically, in more indolent disease. Amyloid arthropathy, which is seen especially in multiple myeloma, can mimic rheumatoid arthritis.

224. A C D

Calcium pyrophosphate dihydrate crystals, which are weakly positively birefringent, are deposited in cartilage and can be seen in joint fluid. Chronic forms of the disease without acute attacks may mimic osteoarthritis, chronic gout, or rheumatoid arthritis. There is no effective prophylactic drug for acute attacks, although nonsteroidal anti-inflammatory drugs can be used.

225. **In a patient suspected of having a connective-tissue disorder, the following findings favour systemic lupus erythematosus:**

A   joint deformities
B   cavitating lung lesion
C   peripheral neuropathy
D   anti-ribonucleoprotein (RNP) antibodies
E   severe Raynaud's phenomenon

226. **Sacroiliitis commonly occurs in the following diseases:**

A   ulcerative colitis
B   Crohn's disease
C   gout
D   ankylosing spondylitis
E   Reiter's syndrome

227. **Polymyalgia rheumatica**

A   is characteristically associated with shoulder girdle muscle wasting
B   is characterised by a positive rheumatoid factor test
C   is invariably 'burnt out' after 2 years
D   is significantly associated with underlying malignancy
E   typically gives rise to raised blood muscle enzyme levels

228. **Avascular necrosis of bone is a recognised complication of**

A   systemic lupus erythematosus
B   renal transplantation
C   sickle cell disease
D   congestive cardiac failure
E   Cushing's syndrome

Answers overleaf

225. NONE CORRECT

Joint deformities are uncommon in SLE, their presence would favour rheumatoid arthritis. A lung cavity and anti-neutrophil cytoplasmic antibodies suggest Wegener's disease; peripheral neuropathy (especially if mononeuritis multiplex), polyarteritis nodosa; RNP antibodies would indicate mixed connective tissue disease and severe Raynaud's, systemic sclerosis or mixed connective tissue disease.

226. A B D E

Sacroiliitis is invariably present in patients with ankylosing spondylitis; HLA-B27 antigen occurs in excess of 95% of these patients. Sacroiliitis is also a feature of inflammatory bowel disease, reactive arthritis, and some types of psoriatic arthritis, especially if the patient possesses the B27 antigen.

227. NONE CORRECT

The muscles involved are painful and stiff but not generally wasted, though wasting can occur due to disuse atrophy. It is now appreciated that the disease can remain active and need steroid therapy for many years in an appreciable percentage of cases. Muscle enzymes, as well as EMG and muscle biopsy are generally normal and unhelpful in diagnosis. The ESR is characteristically 80 mm/hr or more, but by no means invariably so.

228. A B C E

The precise aetiology is unknown and cannot be purely a problem of inadequate blood supply. There are many causes including SLE (though treatment by corticosteroids may be contributory), sickle cell disease and Cushing's syndrome (presumably high corticosteroid output). The immuno-suppressive treatment including prednisolone given to renal transplant patients is also considered causative.

229. Characteristic features of Behcet's disease include

A thrombophlebitis
B glomerulonephritis
C scrotal ulceration
D pyoderma gangrenosum
E myocarditis

230. The following have a recognised association with IgM paraprotein:

A kala-azar
B cold haemagglutinin disease
C chronic lymphatic leukaemia (CLL)
D Waldenstrom's disease
E chronic myeloid leukaemia

231. Extractable nuclear antigens (ENA) are usually found in the following:

A pernicious anaemia
B Sjögren's syndrome
C rheumatoid arthritis
D SLE
E mixed connective tissue disease

232. Characteristic features of non-familial hypogammaglobulinaemia (common variable immunodeficiency) include

A splenomegaly
B bronchiectasis
C pernicious anaemia
D *Giardia lamblia* infestation
E IgA levels are usually greater than IgG and IgM

Answers overleaf

229. A C

Arthritis, anterior uveitis and CNS involvement are other characteristic features. Skin lesions, pustules, papules and erythema nodosum, are common.

230. B C D

No paraproteins are seen in kala-azar, but often there is a massive polyclonal rise in IgM. Cold agglutinin disease, CLL and Waldenstrom's disease are all B-cell lymphoproliferative disorders sometimes associated with an IgM paraprotein, whilst this is not seen in any of the myeloproliferative disorders (see also Q.97 and Q.99).

231. B E

Extractable nuclear antigens are antibodies directed against various cytoplasmic antigens. The commonest are Ro, La, RNP, Scl 70 and Sm. Ro and La are usually present in patients with primary Sjögren's syndrome and RNP typically present in mixed connective tissue disease. Sm is present in only 10% of patients with SLE.

232. A B C D

Lymphoid tissue hyperplasia is a typical finding amongst this group of patients who have the most frequent form of primary immunodeficiency. Recurrent pneumonia (leading to bronchiectasis), sinusitis, otitis media, and gastrointestinal infections are the most frequent infections. There is no marked predisposition to viral infections, and very few suffer from the opportunistic infections seen in patients with AIDS. Secretory and serum IgA levels are virtually absent, IgG and IgM levels being reduced. There is an association with autoimmune disorders.

STATISTICS

233. The following are true:
A the annual prevalence of a condition reflects the number of new cases reported annually
B cohort studies are generally used to study a group of subjects with a particular disease and compare them with normal controls
C in a frequency distribution, the mode is the most frequently observed value
D if a measurement has a skewed distribution, then the mean and mode are always different
E the standard deviation of a population may be smaller than the standard error of a sample mean from that population

234. In the clinical trial of a new treatment
A the null hypothesis is true if there are significant differences between the response of the treatment and placebo group
B the patients should be randomized
C stratum matching of patients is necessary if the groups are small
D in a type one error the null hypothesis is wrongly rejected
E the number of subjects required decreases as the power of the trial increases

235. If a set of values are normally distributed the following are true:
A the median value will be less than the mean
B 2.5% of the values will have numerical values which are smaller than the mean value minus 1.96 standard deviations
C the standard deviation of the values is a measure of how accurately the calculated mean approaches the true population mean
D Student's t-test may be used to compare this set of values with a second set provided they are also normally distributed
E the values may be used to calculate chi-squared

236. The median is used in preference to the arithmetic mean when
A the variance is large
B the sample size is small
C the observations are from a population with a skew distribution
D observer error is likely to be large
E chi-squared is to be calculated

Answers overleaf

233. C D
The **prevalence** of a condition reflects the total number of cases in a population at a given time. **Cohort studies** may be used to study a defined group through time; e.g. a group of subjects exposed to a suspected cause of a disease at a particular time are then followed-up to see whether they develop the disease. The **mode** is the value which occurs most frequently i.e. the maximum value on the frequency distribution curve. If a distribution is positively skewed (long tail on the right side, more large values) it will be less than the mean, if the distribution is negatively skewed (long tail on the left, more small values) it will be greater than the mean. The **standard error of the mean** of a sample (SEM) is a measure of how accurately the true population mean has been estimated. It may be calculated by dividing the standard deviation of the sample by the square root of the sample size ($SD/\sqrt{n}$).

234. B C D
The null hypothesis is rejected if there is a significant difference between the groups. A type I error occurs when the null hypothesis is wrongly rejected (i.e. concluding that a significant difference exists when in reality it does not). A type II error occurs when the null hypothesis is accepted when in reality a genuine difference exists between the two groups. The **power** of a trial is the probability of rejecting the null hypothesis when it is false i.e. of concluding a difference or result of a given size is statistically significant. The power of a trial generally is increased when the number of participants is large and is decreased if the difference to be detected is small.

235. B D
The median value is the value which occurs in the middle when the values are arranged in order of magnitude. For a normal (Gaussian) distribution approximately 68% of the values lie within one standard deviation of the mean and 95.5% within two standard deviations. 1.96 is the 5% percentage point of the normal distribution as 95% of the values lie within 1.96 standard deviations of the mean (2.5% in each tail). The standard deviation is a measure of the spread of a set of values; the SEM measures how accurately the calculated mean approaches the true population mean.

236. C
The median and mode are used in preference to the arithmetic mean when a set of values are from a population with a skewed distribution. In such situations values from the long tail of a skew distribution disproportionately affect the value of the arithmetic mean (average) which may be misleading.

237. **The average heights of two groups of subjects are compared and are stated to be significantly different (p<0.05). The following are true:**
   A   Student's paired test may have been used to calculate p
   B   this result may have arisen by chance alone less than one time in twenty
   C   if the t-test is used the number of degrees of freedom is the total number of observations in both groups minus two
   D   even if the difference is large it has not reached conventional levels of statistical significance
   E   to apply tests of significance validly the groups need to have been chosen randomly

238. **In an assay for serum sodium**
   A   the coefficient of variation of the measurement allows the sensitivity of the assay to be determined
   B   the accuracy of the assay is the degree to which repeated observations conform to each other
   C   the specificity of the assay is a measure of the degree to which other substances may interfere with the serum sodium result
   D   the precision of the assay is a measure of how close the assay result is to the true value
   E   the sensitivity of the assay is the closeness to which the lower limits of the assay approach zero

239. **For the correlation coefficient r, the following are correct:**
   A   the value of r lies between -1 and +1
   B   if r=0.1 this excludes a significant correlation between the variables
   C   if r is negative, one value increases while the other decreases
   D   r would be useful in comparing the relationship between blood pressure and cardiovascular mortality in a population
   E   it can be used to predict one variable from the value of the other

240. **A new antibiotic X is compared with amoxicillin in a clinical trial. A higher proportion of those patients treated with X respond in a given time (chi-squared 4.2; p <0.05). The following are true:**
   A   the improved response to X is clinically significant
   B   treatment with X cannot be worse than treatment with amoxicillin
   C   the results would be invalidated if there was a significant difference in the ages of the two treatment groups
   D   the trial implies that a difference in response of 4.2 times was observed
   E   the results may have occurred by chance one time in twenty

Answers overleaf

237. B C

An **unpaired t-test** would be appropriate since a between group analysis is required. The **paired t-test** is used for within-group comparisons. A **significance value (p)** is the probability that a particular result arose by chance. In small samples the estimate of the mean and standard deviation, etc. are inaccurate. To account for this uncertainty when significance values are calculated we use the **number of degrees of freedom (df)**. The df is the number of independent values which contribute to the calculation of the t-statistic and therefore the significance value. The larger the df the smaller the t-statistic necessary to achieve conventional levels of significance. For a paired t-test this value is the number of observations minus one; in an unpaired t-test it equals the degrees of freedom of both groups which added together equals the total number of observations (in both groups) minus two.

238. C E

The coefficient of variation of the assay is a measure of how often repeated measurements conform to each other; i.e. it reflects the **reproducibility** of the assay. The **accuracy** of an assay reflects the closeness which each measurement has to its true value. If the assay is **specific** then it measures sodium and nothing else. The **precision** of an assay determines how small a change the assay detects.

239. A C

Correlation methods are used to examine whether there is a linear relationship between two continuous variables; the strength of the association is reflected in the value of r (-1 to +1). If the correlation is strong r has values of less than -0.5 or greater than +0.5. The statistical significance of a particular r is calculated separately (NB even if a correlation is poor, it may still be statistically significant). Although two variables may be correlated, this does not allow a value for one variable to be calculated from a value of the second. **Regression analysis** and the derivation of a regression equation may be used to calculate the value of one (dependent) variable from a second (independent) variable. Mortality is not a continuous variable.

240. C E

Statistical significance does not imply clinical significance. In addition to assessing the clinical improvement produced by a therapy, account must also be taken of side effects. **Chi-squared** is a calculated statistic used to compare proportions and has no immediate intuitive meaning unlike a p-value or a mean. Any bias or confounding element (e.g. differences in the severity of disease between the two groups) may invalidate a trial.

1. In the heart

A the pulmonary valve is normally bicuspid
B the right bundle of His divides into anterior and posterior hemibundles
C the coronary sinus opens into the right atrium
D blood leaving the coronary sinus is less de-oxygenated than the atrial blood into which it drains
E the S-A node lies in the anterior wall of the left atrium

2. A plasma bicarbonate level of 34 mmol/l would be an unexpected finding in a patient with

A Conn's syndrome
B vomiting due to pyloric stenosis
C untreated diabetic ketoacidosis
D chronic cor pulmonale
E chronic renal failure

3. A high plasma inorganic phosphate level is a characteristic finding in

A diabetic ketoacidosis
B the osteodystrophy of chronic renal failure
C hypoparathyroidism
D nutritional rickets
E Paget's disease

4. A low plasma sodium (as measured by the auto-analyser) may be a consequence of

A alcoholic cirrhosis
B salt depletion
C hyperlipidaemia
D Cushing's syndrome
E hyperglycaemia

121

5. **In hypertrophic cardiomyopathy**

    A   atrial fibrillation indicates a poor prognosis
    B   the characteristic murmur is typically loudest in the aortic area
    C   a diastolic murmur is present in the majority of cases
    D   trinitrin reduces outflow obstruction
    E   there are characteristic echocardiographic findings

6. **The following statements are correct:**

    A   complete heart block is associated with a poor prognosis in anterior myocardial infarction
    B   complete heart block complicating myocardial infarction characteristically resolves if the patient survives
    C   the A-V node is supplied by the circumflex coronary artery in 90% of patients
    D   acute mitral regurgitation associated with myocardial infarction can be easily distinguished from rheumatic mitral regurgitation by the site of the murmur
    E   the commonest cause of chronic complete heart block is ischaemic heart disease

7. **Systemic blood pressure is increased**

    A   on the assumption of the upright from the supine position
    B   on sudden exposure to cold
    C   always when heart rate increases
    D   by brain stem asphyxia
    E   in response to stimulation of peripheral chemoreceptors

8. **Isolated calcific aortic stenosis in the elderly**

    A   is rheumatic in origin in the majority of cases
    B   may present as congestive cardiac failure
    C   is associated characteristically with a systolic ejection click
    D   tends to soften and delay the aortic component of the second sound
    E   is not haemodynamically important in the absence of a thrill

9. **A rumbling apical diastolic murmur is a recognised finding in**

   A   systemic arterial hypertension
   B   thyrotoxicosis
   C   mitral regurgitation
   D   complete heart block
   E   ventricular septal defect

10. **Intracellular inclusion bodies are seen in the following conditions:**

    A   Alzheimer's disease
    B   rabies
    C   sarcoidosis
    D   yellow fever
    E   cytomegalovirus infection

11. **The following drugs may have a causative association with the following renal diseases:**

    A   tetracycline and uraemia
    B   penicillamine and papillary necrosis
    C   allopurinol and uric acid nephropathy
    D   gold and heavy proteinuria
    E   procainamide and glomerulonephritis

12. **Adverse effects of sulphasalazine include**

    A   diarrhoea
    B   haemolytic anaemia
    C   folate deficiency
    D   male erectile impotence
    E   headaches

13. The following drug combinations are usually undesirable:

A   digoxin and amiodarone
B   metoclopramide and chlorpromazine
C   cholestyramine and prednisolone
D   levodopa and nifedipine
E   ranitidine and metronidazole

14. Phenothiazines may cause

A   agranulocytosis
B   photosensitivity
C   increased lacrimation
D   priapism
E   cholestatic jaundice

15. Morphine

A   is mainly excreted unchanged by the kidneys
B   produces mydriasis
C   decreases intestinal smooth muscle tone
D   decreases peripheral venous capacitance
E   is antagonised by naloxone

16. Exfoliative dermatitis

A   may contribute to heart failure
B   gives hyperpyrexia
C   with pruritus indicates a lymphoma
D   can complicate psoriasis
E   may be responsible for lymphadenopathy

17. In patients with non-metastatic manifestations of malignancy

A hypercalcaemia may be suppressed by prednisolone
B thyrotoxicosis associated with chorioncarcinoma does not show eye signs
C the commonest tumour to cause polycythaemia is the hypernephroma
D ectopic ADH (vasopressin) secretion presents with hypokalaemia
E myasthenia responding to neostigmine is found in association with bronchial carcinoma

18. In insulin dependent diabetes (IDDM)

A persistence of islet cell antibodies increases the likelihood of associated autoimmune disease
B there is an increased incidence of HLA B8 status
C there is 90% concordance in identical twins
D a history of recent mumps virus infection is common at presentation
E retinopathy is usually present at diagnosis

19. In primary hyperparathyroidism there is

A an invariable increase in the level of parathyroid hormone in blood
B an increase in tubular reabsorption of calcium in the presence of hypercalciuria
C the possibility of hypocalcaemic tetany in a neonate whose mother has the condition
D a single adenoma in about 40% of cases
E a recognised association with systemic arterial hypertension

20. Non-secreting adenomas of the pituitary gland

A are composed entirely of chromophobe cells
B rarely cause expansion of the pituitary fossa
C rarely give rise to pituitary failure
D are a recognised association in patients with primary hyperparathyroidism due to hyperplasia of the parathyroid glands
E may progress to involve the supraopticohypophyseal tract thereby causing diabetes insipidus

21. **In Crohn's disease**

    A   approximately one third of patients will require surgery
    B   azathioprine's main role is steroid sparing
    C   acute phase protein concentrations are more likely to be elevated in small bowel disease
    D   the most important long term adverse effect of continued corticosteroid therapy is diabetes
    E   perianal involvement often responds to metronidazole

22. **In acute pancreatitis**

    A   urgent ultrasound is required if the patient is jaundiced
    B   emergency ERCP is needed to confirm the diagnosis
    C   pancreatic pseudo-cyst is a likely cause of persistent hyper-amylasaemia
    D   progression to chronic pancreatitis is common
    E   hypercalcaemia may follow the acute presentation

23. **Concerning oesophageal chest pain**

    A   it can cause exercise induced chest pain
    B   the acid provocation test is obsolete
    C   the most useful test is 24 hour pH monitoring
    D   a positive response to nitrates excludes the oesophagus as the cause of chest pain
    E   acid reflux can lead to oesophageal spasm

24. **The following are true statements concerning carcinoid tumours and the carcinoid syndrome:**

    A   the commonest primary site is the jejunum
    B   with a small bowel primary tumour, the development of the carcinoid syndrome implies liver metastases
    C   left sided cardiac lesions do not occur
    D   high volume secretory diarrhoea may occur
    E   tumours are most commonly incidental findings

25. **The following drugs are safe to use in combination with warfarin:**

    A ranitidine
    B co-trimoxazole
    C carbamazepine
    D ibuprofen
    E salbutamol

26. **An adult has taken 50 aspirin tablets; after four hours**

    A coma is to be expected
    B gastric lavage is of no value
    C alkaline diuresis is the treatment of choice
    D peritoneal dialysis could be of value therapeutically
    E hypoglycaemia may be present

27. **Features of sickle cell anaemia in adults include**

    A leg ulcers
    B aseptic bone necrosis
    C dysphagia
    D priapism
    E nocturia

28. **In multiple myeloma**

    A radiotherapy is a useful means of controlling hypercalcaemia
    B the prognosis is closely correlated with renal function
    C hyperviscosity is more common in IgA than IgG types
    D peripheral neuropathy is a recognised complication
    E the serum alkaline phosphatase is characteristically normal

29. The following are causes of a leuco-erythroblastic blood picture:

A carcinomatosis
B respiratory distress in neonates
C septicaemia
D myelofibrosis
E severe untreated pernicious anaemia

30. The following organisms are recognised causes of pneumonia:

A *Chlamydia pneumoniae*
B *Mycoplasma hominis*
C *Chlamydia trachomatis*
D *Streptococcus pyogenes*
E *Legionella pneumophila*

31. In the diagnosis of typhoid

A the Widal test is useful
B leucopenia supports the diagnosis
C bone marrow aspiration has the highest yield for culturing *S. typhi*
D stool cultures are always negative in the first week
E rose spots are a reliable sign

32. The following are true:

A measuring maternal serum alpha fetoprotein (AFP) is useful in assessing the risk of a fetus having Down's syndrome
B over 50% of spontaneous first trimester abortions are the result of fetal chromosomal abnormalities
C fetal blood samples are necessary if a pre-natal diagnosis of haemophilia A is to be made
D chorionic villus sampling allows fetal cystic fibrosis to be diagnosed in the first trimester
E amniocentesis allows all fetal chromosomal abnormalities to be identified

33. **The following are recognised findings in osteogenesis imperfecta:**

A blue sclerae
B otosclerosis
C pathological fracture
D low alkaline phosphatase
E partial remission in the female reproductive years

34. **The following statements are true of attacks of acute intermittent porphyria (AIP):**

A Ehrlich's aldehyde reagent is of value in diagnosis
B postural hypotension is a characteristic finding
C pain in the limbs is a characteristic complaint
D diazepam is a typical precipitant
E carbohydrate infusions are of value in management

35. **Recognised features of carotid artery disease include**

A diplopia
B transient ipsilateral monocular blindness
C vertigo
D ptosis
E miosis

36. **The following restrictions with respect to driving apply to patients at risk of having seizures:**

A patients are obliged to contact the DVLC if they believe themselves to be at risk of seizures
B a patient's doctor is obliged to inform the DVLC of a patient at risk of seizures
C a patient may continue to drive following a single nocturnal seizure
D a recent diagnosis of cerebral glioma prohibits driving
E a recent diagnosis of bronchogenic carcinoma prohibits driving

37. **In the chronic fatigue syndrome**

    A   previous psychiatric illness is a recognised risk factor
    B   a mild rise in creatine phosphokinase is commonly detected
    C   persistent viral antigen is detected in a minority of patients
    D   decreased physical activity is a risk factor for the continuation of fatigue
    E   the majority of affected patients fulfill psychiatric criteria for depression

38. **In patients affected with HIV-1 related dementia**

    A   dementia may be the presenting feature
    B   language disturbance and visuoconstructive difficulties are early features of the dementia
    C   intracerebral Kaposi's sarcoma is rarely the cause of dementia
    D   *Cryptococcus* is the most common opportunistic cause of dementia
    E   the majority of demented patients have a raised CSF protein

39. **Benign intracranial hypertension is typically associated with**

    A   enlarged blind spots
    B   reduced visual acuity
    C   a presentation in the puerperium
    D   mild elevation of the CSF protein
    E   sixth nerve palsy

40. **A patient presents with a painful red eye. The following findings are more suggestive of anterior uveitis than acute conjunctivitis:**

    A   blurring of vision
    B   profuse discharge
    C   small pupil
    D   photophobia
    E   clear media

41. A shift in the haemoglobin/oxygen dissociation curve to the right

A means that for a given pO_2 there is less oxygen per gram of haemoglobin
B occurs in anaemia
C occurs when the pCO_2 is increased
D could result from an increased concentration of 2,3 diphospho-glycerate in the erythrocytes
E is favoured by a fall in temperature

42. Breast development in a five-year-old girl

A may be due to an arrhenoblastoma of the ovary
B frequently has no identifiable organic cause
C is a common result of XXY chromosomal constitution
D requires urgent laparotomy to examine the ovaries
E may be a late result of maternal oestrogens transferred before birth

43. Recognised causes of stridor include

A foreign body in the left main bronchus
B *Haemophilus influenzae* infection
C vascular ring
D hypercalcaemia
E *C. diphtheriae* infection

44. An acute confusional state is

A often responsive to tricyclic antidepressant drug therapy
B a characteristic feature of myxoedema
C characterised by loss of memory for recent events
D typically reversible
E more common with pre-existing brain disease

45. Hysterical amnesia

A typically is a patchy loss of memory
B typically resolves within 48 hours
C is a conscious reaction
D has a recognised association with head injury
E is usually provoked by stress

46. The following are recognised features of schizophrenia:

A disorientation in time
B incongruity of affect
C suspiciousness
D perseveration
E hearing one's own thoughts spoken aloud

47. Recognised features of renal amyloid deposition are

A monoclonal gammopathy
B histology showing intra-glomerular and tubular staining with Sudan black
C heavy proteinuria
D occurs as a long-term complication of haemodialysis
E serum amyloid P component (SAP) scan allows assessment of the extent of systemic deposition

48. The following are true statements:

A angiotensin converting-enzyme inhibitors should never be prescribed in cases of renovascular hypertension
B renal failure is the commonest cause of death in non-insulin dependent diabetes
C in IgA nephropathy (Berger's disease) haematuria typically follows 2–3 weeks after an upper respiratory tract infection
D a transplanted renal allograft will function provided donor warm ischaemic time is kept below 2 hours
E in chronic reflux nephropathy there is usually a history of previous recurrent urinary infection

49. **On chest X-ray the upper zone is more commonly affected than the lower zone in**

    A   asbestosis
    B   silicosis
    C   cryptogenic fibrosing alveolitis
    D   ankylosing spondylitis
    E   systemic sclerosis

50. **Recognised causes of pulmonary eosinophilia (chest X-ray shadowing and peripheral blood eosinophilia) include**

    A   *Ascaris lumbricoides* infestation
    B   systemic lupus erythematosus
    C   sarcoidosis
    D   polyarteritis nodosa
    E   cryptogenic fibrosing alveolitis

51. **In the obstructive sleep apnoea syndrome**

    A   complete obstruction typically occurs during non-REM sleep
    B   there is an association with obesity and hypertension
    C   oximetry alone is a useful screening procedure
    D   sustained pulmonary hypertension is a rare occurrence
    E   tracheostomy is the definitive treatment

52. **The following are typical features of reactive arthritis:**

    A   onset after *E. coli* enteritis
    B   presence of viable organisms within the joint
    C   asymmetric lower limb joint involvement
    D   episcleritis
    E   Achilles tendonitis

53. **D-Penicillamine therapy in rheumatoid arthritis may**

    A induce a lupus-like syndrome
    B lower rheumatoid factor titres
    C cause Goodpasture's syndrome
    D produce ageusia (altered taste sensation)
    E cause malabsorption

54. **The following are often desirable when carrying out a clinical trial of a new drug:**

    A apparatus with which to make reproducible observations
    B use of a double blind cross-over method
    C administration of the drug to patients undergoing treatment with other drugs
    D the drug should have been tested extensively in animals
    E a pilot study

55. **Recognised side-effects of lithium carbonate include**

    A polyuria
    B hypopituitarism
    C diarrhoea
    D intention tremor
    E hypothyroidism

56. **The following are features of atropine poisoning:**

    A fever
    B bradycardia
    C profuse sweating
    D pin-point pupils
    E hallucinations

57. **The following are poor prognostic signs in a patient with *Neisseria meningitidis* infection:**

    A   absence of neck stiffness
    B   widespread ecchymosis
    C   CSF protein >2.5 g/l
    D   leucopenia
    E   a skin/rectal temperature difference of >3°C

58. **Tuberculosis of the respiratory tract may cause**

    A   wheezing
    B   ARDS
    C   pleural effusion
    D   unilateral hilar lymphadenopathy
    E   massive haemoptysis

59. **The following diseases can be diagnosed by examination of a blood film:**

    A   rat-bite fever
    B   relapsing fever
    C   Lyme disease
    D   African trypanosomiasis
    E   Oroya fever

60. **Amoebic liver abscess is commonly associated with**

    A   jaundice
    B   splenomegaly
    C   dysentery
    D   pericarditis
    E   raised hemidiaphragm

PRACTICE EXAM ANSWERS

1. **C**

   The pulmonary valve is normally tricuspid like the aortic valve. It is the left bundle of His which is described as dividing into anterior and posterior hemibundles or fascicles. The heart is remarkable in that a high proportion of oxygen is extracted from the coronary blood, and so the blood returning from the coronary sinus into the right atrium between the inferior caval opening and the right atrioventricular valve is highly de-oxygenated. Therefore increased oxygen delivery is produced by increased coronary flow rather than increased oxygen extraction. The sino-atrial node lies high in the wall of the right atrium near its junction with the superior vena cava.

2. **C E**

   The metabolic acidosis of uraemia and diabetic ketoacidosis would make a high plasma bicarbonate an extremely unlikely occurrence. Most causes of hypokalaemia, including Conn's syndrome, are associated with a metabolic alkalosis which can be gross in pyloric stenosis. In chronic cor pulmonale, a raised bicarbonate level would indicate renal compensation of a respiratory acidosis due to CO_2 retention.

3. **A B C**

   Phosphate (like potassium) is predominantly an intracellular ion and this may be reflected by an increased extracellular fluid concentration in the presence of acidosis, due to cell membrane dysfunction. Hyperphosphataemia is believed to play an aetiological role in renal osteodystrophy by leading to secondary (and tertiary) hyperparathyroidism. The plasma phosphate is typically low in all vitamin D deficiency related bone disease. It is normal in uncomplicated Paget's disease.

4. **A B C E**

   ADH released by blood volume contraction contributes to the hyponatraemia of salt depletion and hyperglycaemia. Also, in dehydration, increased proximal tubular reabsorption limits the volume of fluid reaching the diluting segment of the distal tubule and hence water excretion. Oat cell lung cancers may secrete ADH. In hyperglycaemia, osmotically active solute in the blood also contributes to hyponatraemia. ADH is also released inappropriately in cirrhosis of the liver where hypoproteinaemia will also contribute to the redistribution of salt and water as interstitial oedema. In hyperlipidaemia, hyponatraemia is more apparent then real, due to plasma water being replaced by sodium-free lipid (see Q.147).

5. **A E**

The development of atrial fibrillation or identification of ventricular tachycardia indicates a poor prognosis. The clinical findings are usually of left ventricular hypertrophy, a long ejection systolic murmur at the left sternal edge due to outflow obstruction, and often some mitral regurgitation. However, significant myopathy may be present without outflow gradient when no murmur may be apparent. If in sinus rhythm a loud fourth heart sound is present. A third heart sound is common but a diastolic murmur is uncommon and would indicate mixed aortic valve disease. Outflow obstruction is liable to increase with trinitrin as this reduces ventricular volume and also lowers arterial pressure. The echo shows combinations of asymmetric septal hypertrophy (ASH), systolic anterior motion of the mitral apparatus (SAM), a high ejection fraction with early closure of the aortic valve, and an outflow gradient which can be measured by Doppler.

6. **A B**

Complete and lesser degrees of A-V block are more common with inferior myocardial infarcts and characteristically resolve. This is probably related to the fact that the A-V node and bundle of His are supplied by the right coronary artery in about 90% of cases. When complete heart block occurs with anterior infarcts it usually indicates massive necrosis; hence the poor prognosis, which is mainly related to the poor left ventricular function and severe coronary disease. However, if residual complete or incomplete atrio-ventricular block or peripheral blocks persist, consideration should be given to a permanent pacemaker. An echo usually elucidates the cause of mitral reflux and is useful to distinguish it from an acute VSD in infarction. Chronic complete heart block is often due to conduction tissue fibrosis, either idiopathic sclerosis (Lenegre's disease) or fibrocalcific degeneration (Lev's disease), without clinically important ischaemic disease (see also Q.20).

7. **B D E**

The blood pressure may be calculated by the following equation:

Blood pressure = Cardiac Output × Peripheral Resistance

Therefore, it rises when peripheral resistance increases on exposure to cold – this is sometimes used as a 'cold pressor' test. It falls when venous return and hence cardiac output falls, and a transient drop of blood pressure on rising may be seen in normal subjects but this should not persist. It does not necessarily increase when the heart rate increases, as an increased heart rate does not necessarily produce an increase in cardiac output. Stimulation of the peripheral chemoreceptors and hypoxia itself act on the pressor area in the medulla to give an increase in blood pressure.

8. **B D**

    The majority of cases are secondary to bicuspid valves or to non-rheumatic calcification of a tricuspid aortic valve seen in the very old. The presence of mitral valve disease or significant aortic regurgitation would suggest a rheumatic origin. A relatively quiet murmur may be present with severe disease, particularly if the patient is in heart failure or has emphysema; severe disease is suggested by an aortic systolic thrill. Elderly patients may present with cardiac failure rather than classically with dyspnoea, angina or syncope. Significant aortic stenosis prolongs left ventricular ejection time but this is often difficult to appreciate. A click is unusual in clinically significant calcific disease.

9. **B C E**

    A fourth heart sound is usual in hypertension. A murmur mimicking mitral stenosis may occur when there is a greatly increased flow across a normal mitral valve in mitral regurgitation, VSD, patent ductus and occasionally in thyrotoxicosis and other hyperdynamic circulatory conditions. Similar murmurs occur in aortic regurgitation (Austin Flint), acute rheumatic fever (Carey Coombs) and with atrial myxomas. The murmur of tricuspid stenosis and tricuspid flow murmurs may occasionally be heard at the apex. Complete heart block usually presents with an ejection systolic murmur due to a large stroke volume.

10. **B E**

    Intracellular inclusion bodies are an histological feature of certain viral infections. In rabies the Negri bodies are accumulations of viral RNA and are seen in the hippocampus and cerebellar Purkinje cells. 'Owls eye' inclusions are seen in parotid, liver, lung and kidney in CMV infections. The Councilman bodies demonstrable in the liver in yellow fever are not inclusions but eosinophilic necrotic cells and these are present in other forms of hepatitis. Although an infectious aetiology has been postulated in Alzheimer's disease evidence suggests that non-viral agents could be implicated (see Q.126).

11. A D

The tetracyclines (except doxycycline) can aggravate uraemia dangerously and should be avoided in patients with anything other than minimal renal impairment (see also Q. 35). Penicillamine, like gold, produces an immune-complex membranous glomerulonephritis, usually presenting with proteinuria. Although procainamide is often responsible for a lupus syndrome, glomerulonephritis is unusual in drug-induced SLE (see Q.222).

12. A B E

Sulphasalazine comprises sulphapyridine and 5-aminosalicylic acid. The former produces nausea, rashes, headaches, oxidative haemolysis and a reversible reduction in sperm count. The latter has been associated with diarrhoea and renal impairment (see also Q.81).

13. A B C D

Pharmacodynamic interactions between drugs having similar or opposite effects are common and often predictable. Metoclopramide and chlorpromazine, both dopamine antagonists, increase the risk of extrapyramidal adverse effects. Levodopa and nifedipine summate their hypotensive effects.

14. A B D E

Other clinically important side-effects of phenothiazine therapy include orthostatic hypotension and the extra-pyramidal syndromes.

15. E

Morphine is detoxicated mainly by conjugation with glucuronic acid in the liver and should be used with caution in cirrhosis. Pin-point pupils (severe miosis) are an important sign of intoxication or addiction with opiates. Intestinal smooth muscle tone is increased and propulsive waves diminished, explaining the constipating effects of these drugs. The therapeutic effect of morphine in acute left ventricular failure is probably largely due to its venodilating action.

16. A D E

Exfoliative dermatitis (erythroderma) will contribute to congestive cardiac failure by virtue of the increased blood flow in the skin, a factor also tending to *hypo*- not *hyper*thermia. Pruritus is common and not indicative of an underlying lymphoma. Psoriasis is responsible for about 25% of cases of exfoliative dermatitis. Lymphadenopathy is often marked with exfoliative dermatitis, constituting so-called dermatopathic lymphadenopathy.

17. A B C

The non-metastatic hypercalcaemia of malignancy cannot always be shown to be due to excess parathormone-like activity and in at least half the cases, responds to steroids. Human chorionic thyrotrophin found in the normal placenta and in chorioncarcinomas does not cause eye signs. Hypernephroma is a more frequent cause of polycythaemia than phaeochromocytoma, cerebellar haemangiomata, uterine myomata and hepatomas. Ectopic ADH secretion presents with hyponatraemia and symptoms attributed to cerebral oedema. The myasthenic syndrome of malignancy (Eaton-Lambert) differs from classical myasthenia gravis in several respects including little or no response to neostigmine. Guanidine hydrochloride improves muscle strength in many of these patients.

18. A B

Islet cell antibodies are present in over 90% of patients with IDDM (Type 1 diabetes) at presentation. 20 years after diagnosis, only 10% of patients retain islet cell antibodies and these patients are more likely to have other organ-specific autoimmune disease (Type 1b diabetes). Several HLA types have been found with increased frequency in patients with IDDM, including DR3, DR4, B8 and B15. Twin studies indicate a much lower concordance in type 1 compared to type 2 diabetes. Although there have been 'outbreaks' of diabetes associated with viral infection, this remains uncommon. In contrast to NIDDM complications of any form are rare at presentation in IDDM.

19. B C E

The hypercalcaemia of hyperparathyroidism is often associated with raised parathyroid hormone (PTH) levels. A PTH level within the normal range however, is abnormal in the presence of hypercalcaemia, as the raised calcium should inhibit PTH. This occurs in the other causes of hypercalcaemia such as sarcoidosis. Hypercalciuria is not as great as would be predicted from other causes of hypercalcaemia, as there is increased renal tubular absorption of calcium. Foetal parathyroid activity may be suppressed by maternal hypercalcaemia, resulting in tetany in the neonate. A third of patients have hypertension, in part due to renal damage, but in some, recovering when hypercalcaemia is corrected. Over 80% of patients have a solitary adenoma, 15% have diffuse hyperplasia, and a small minority a carcinoma of one gland.

20. D

Although chromophobe cells were previously thought to be nonsecretory, direct immunostaining for pituitary hormones has indicated that many produce hormones, particularly prolactin. Radiological evidence of pituitary fossa expansion is present in over 90% of patients and extension of the tumour to involve optic chiasm and nerves, the 3rd, 4th and 6th cranial nerves and hypothalamus may occur. Destruction of normal pituitary tissue by the expanding tumour typically leads to a sequence of anterior pituitary deficits: growth hormone, gonadotrophins, corticotrophin then thyrotrophin. Diabetes insipidus due to supraoptico-hypophyseal tract involvement is rare. There is an association with parathyroid hyperplasia or adenoma (MEN type 1) (see also Q.56 and Q.152).

21. B E

Nearly 75% of patients with Crohn's disease require surgery at some time in their lives. The earlier the surgery is in the history the more likely is the need for repeated surgery. Corticosteroid usage is predominantly short term to induce remissions. A small number (5–10%) of patients become steroid dependent. The major metabolic problem with this latter group is osteoporosis, and azathioprine has a useful steroid-sparing role in these patients. Acute phase protein responses are higher in large bowel disease.

22. A C

Acute pancreatitis still has an appreciable mortality (up to 10%). The commonest associated factor is biliary tract stones if the patient has jaundice. An emergency ultrasound followed by an ERCP and sphincterotomy is indicated. Injecting dye into the pancreatic duct at ERCP may be dangerous. Most causes of acute pancreatitis do not go on to chronic pancreatitis. Persistent pain and hyperamylasaemia suggest a complication like pseudocyst or abscess. Some patients can become profoundly hypocalcaemic (see also Q.84).

23. **A E**

Oesophageal chest pain can exactly mimic angina pain including a response to nitrates. Altered oesophageal motility may be secondary to oesophageal reflux or to a motility disorder. The (Bernstein) acid provocation test still has a role as has 24 hour pH monitoring. Motility disorders require oesophageal manometry.

24. **B D E**

The commonest site for a primary carcinoid tumour, often discovered incidentally, is the ileum. With carcinoids of the gut, liver involvement (metastases) is necessary before the syndrome is said to occur. Right-sided valvular lesions (tricuspid and pulmonary stenosis and incompetence) are well described (see Q.9). However, the rarer bronchial carcinoids can result in a carcinoid syndrome in the absence of metastatic disease and they are also associated with left-sided cardiac valvular lesions. The tumour can produce a number of hormones e.g. VIP, and a high volume secretory diarrhoea may result.

25. **A D E**

The main interactions with warfarin are due either to hepatic enzyme inhibition e.g. cimetidine, cotrimoxazole, or to enzyme induction e.g. anticoagulants, rifampicin, phenytoin (see also Q.36). Non-steroidal anti-inflammatory drugs may predispose to gastric erosion and ulceration, with consequent risk of G.I. bleeding.

26. **C D E**

Salicylate is secreted into the stomach long after ingestion. A respiratory alkalosis is the commonest metabolic abnormality in adults, but is only transient in children who develop metabolic acidosis more readily. Although peritoneal dialysis removes salicylate effectively, it is not used unless an alkaline diuresis is not possible. Salicylates impair carbohydrate metabolism.

27. **A B D E**

    Infection of bone infarcts occurs and tends to be with salmonella. Other problems of the adult sickler include severe anaemia, crises, pulmonary infarcts, gallstones, cerebrovascular complications and recurrent haematuria.

28. **B C D E**

    Radiotherapy is only useful for bone pain in myeloma. Poor renal function is closely correlated with a poor prognosis. Hyperviscosity occurs in IgA myeloma due to polymerisation of paraprotein molecules. Polyneuropathy occurs due to amyloidosis, or it may be of unknown aetiology as with carcinoma.

29. **A B C D E**

    All can cause leuco-erythroblastic anaemia. This is merely a descriptive term for the presence of immature red and white cells in the peripheral blood, and does not imply aetiology.

30. **A C D E**

    Three types of *Chlamydia* can cause pneumonia: *C. psittaci, C. pneumoniae* and *C. trachomatis*. The latter occurs in children infected at birth, 2–6 weeks after delivery. *Legionella pneumophila* is the commonest of the legionellas to cause pneumonia but remember other legionellas can also cause pneumonia. *Mycoplasma pneumoniae*, not *Mycoplasma hominis*, causes pneumonia.

31. **B C E**

    Bone marrow aspiration recovers *S. typhi* in 90% of patients which compares to 75% from blood cultures. The Widal test is a poor diagnostic test because of cross-reactivity with other *Salmonella* and past immunisation. Although classically *S. typhi* is absent from the stools in the first week this is not invariable and a stool culture should always be performed when a patient with suspected typhoid is admitted to hospital.

32. **A B D E**

    The maternal AFP is often lower than normal in mothers carrying a fetus with Down's syndrome; a low maternal AFP in combination with maternal age is a more sensitive method of identifying preganancies with a high risk of an affected fetus, than maternal age alone.

Although chorionic villus sampling (CVS), performed between 9 and 12 weeks gestation, carries a 1–2% risk of miscarriage, it allows first trimester diagnosis of many single gene defects using DNA analysis. Cultured cells allow many inherited metabolic defects and all chromosomal abnormalities to be detected. After 16–18 weeks cultured amniotic cells obtained by amniocentesis becomes the method of choice. Fetal blood sampling is no longer necessary to diagnose fetal haemophilia and is only used to confirm the results obtained by other methods, and for rapid chromosomal analysis.

33. **A B C E**

Osteogenesis imperfecta, in which there appears to be a generalised defect in the maturation of collagen, manifests in the eye (blue sclerae), ear (otosclerosis), skeleton (multiple fractures), loose jointedness and in skin. The alkaline phosphatase is normal or perhaps raised following a fracture. There is said to be a partial remission from pathological fractures during the reproductive years in women presumably owing to the effects of oestrogen. A low alkaline phosphatase is characteristic of hypophosphatasia, a rare inherited syndrome of short stature, which usually presents as rickets.

34. **A B C E**

Porphobilinogen excreted in large amounts in the urine in acute attacks gives a red colour with Ehrlich's reagent which is not extractable with chloroform (cf. urobilinogen and indoles). Labile hypertension, postural hypotension, tachycardia and neuritic limb pains are attributed to autonomic and peripheral nervous system dysfunction. Classical precipitant drugs include barbiturates, anticonvulsants, oral contraceptives and sulphonamides. Glucose infusions often help to abort acute attacks but hypotonic fluid must be used with extreme caution because of the risk of inappropriate ADH secretion (SIADH) in this condition (see Q.40).

35. **B D E**

Diplopia and vertigo are features of vertebral and basilar artery disease. Ipsilateral blindness is caused by embolisation of the ophthalmic artery. Sympathetic nerve damage due to carotid artery occlusion or dissection may cause ptosis and miosis.

36. A D E

The patient but not his or her doctor is obliged to contact the DVLC, although it is sensible practice to record in the case notes that a patient has been counselled about driving. Patients must be free from any attack for two years or have had only attacks whilst asleep for three years before driving is permitted. A diagnosis of primary malignant cerebral tumour, cerebral metastasis or even bronchogenic carcinoma without cerebral metastasis is associated with such a high risk of a seizure that driving is prohibited.

37. A C D E

Few risk factors have been identified for the chronic fatigue syndrome apart from previous psychiatric illness. More than 75% of affected patients have a concurrent psychiatric illness, depression being present in more than half. No relationship has been demonstrated between clinical status and any laboratory findings. The treatment of choice appears to be a gentle return to physical activity and treatment of the associated depression, usually with a tricyclic antidepressant.

38. A C E

HIV-1 virus related dementia eventually affects 70–90% of patients with AIDS and may be the presenting feature. Patients present with apathy, depression and irritability. Features of cortical dysfunction, such as aphasia and visuoconstructive difficulties, are late manifestations. Toxoplasmosis is the most common opportunistic cause of dementia (see also Q.93).

39. A E

In benign intracranial hypertension investigations including CSF protein levels are normal. Signs reflect the raised intracranial pressure (sixth nerve palsy) and papilloedema (enlarged blind spots). Acuity is not normally affected unless papilloedema extends to affect the macula. The combination of a blurred optic disc and reduced visual acuity suggests papillitis. Presentation in the puerperium, after infection or dehydration, suggests venous sinus thrombosis and urgent consideration of anticoagulation.

40. A C D

Other causes of a 'red eye' are subconjunctival haemorrhage, which is not painful, and acute closed-angle glaucoma and keratitis which are. With conjunctival injection, the vessels fade from fornix to limbus, and move with the conjunctiva. Ciliary vessel injection with intraocular inflammation gives the reverse findings (see also Q.169).

41. A C D

The oxygen dissociation curve is usually plotted as the percentage saturation of haemoglobin with oxygen against oxygen tension. A shift to the right means that for a given oxygen tension there is reduced saturation of haemoglobin with oxygen. This shift can be brought about by increases in hydrogen ion concentration, in pCO_2 and 2,3 diphosphoglycerate. The dissociation curve applies in anaemia even though the oxygen capacity is low.

42. B

Arrhenoblastoma of the ovary is a very rare tumour, almost confined to adults, and causes androgen (not oestrogen) secretion. Breast development is frequently the first manifestation of constitutional precocious puberty in a girl, with no recognisable organic changes. (It follows, therefore, that laparotomy to examine the ovaries is rarely necessary.) The XXY chromosome constitution (Klinefelter's syndrome) results in a phenotypic male and gynaecomastia occurs at or after the usual time of puberty. Maternal oestrogens frequently cause breast enlargement in newborn babies, both male and female, but this disappears within 2–3 weeks of birth (see also Q.62).

43. B C E

A foreign body in a main bronchus may cause initial spluttering and coughing when first inhaled, but will then probably be silent until infection or lung collapse occur. *Haemophilus influenzae* is a frequent secondary invader in acute laryngotracheitis, which causes marked stridor. A vascular ring round the trachea may cause definite, though rather faint stridor, and *C. diphtheriae* will cause stridor by infection of fauces or larynx.

44. C D E

Almost every disease, bodily insult and drug has been credited with precipitating acute confusion. Commonly implicated factors are trauma, surgery, heart failure, infection, anoxia and sedative drugs. Confusion is not, however, a characteristic feature of myxoedema. Senile dementia is a very common predisposing condition and tricyclics may precipitate a confusional state. Phenothiazines such as thioridazine may be used therapeutically but dealing with the precipitating factor is most important.

45. A B D E

When amnesia is of hysterical origin, rather than due to some organic cause, emotionally charged events may be forgotten, whilst memory for other events taking place at the same time may be retained. The majority of such states resolve quickly as the situation which produced them alters. The symptoms are of unconscious, rather than conscious origin. The reaction can follow traumatic events, in particular head injury, and can be provoked by physical or psychological stress. If no stress can be found even after interviewing an informant, the diagnosis of hysterical amnesia should be doubted.

46. B C E

The most frequently occurring symptoms of acute schizophrenia are lack of insight, auditory hallucinations, ideas of reference, suspiciousness, flatness of mood, voices speaking to the patient, persecutory delusions, and hearing one's own thoughts spoken aloud. The commonest forms of hallucinations are auditory, but visual, tactile, olfactory and somatic are recognised. The patient is usually fully orientated. Perseveration is the persistent and in-appropriate repetition of the same word and thoughts, and is a recognised feature of dementia. There are three common changes in mood; patients can be irritable, anxious, depressed or elated; they can show a flattening of mood; they can display incongruity of affect (an inappropriate mood state) (see Q.193).

47. A C E

Deposition of amyloid protein within the kidneys may occur in primary amyloidosis or as a result of conditions involving chronic suppuration or inflammation, disorders of plasma cell function and with hereditary amyloid (familial Mediterranean fever). A nephrotic presentation is common and the classical histological staining is with Congo red (apple-green birefringence is seen under polarised light). The recently developed SAP scan utilises serum amyloid P component, a normal plasma constituent, which binds to amyloid fibrils – I^{123} radiolabelled SAP is injected and localises to amyloid present in any region of the body. The amyloid protein that accumulates in dialysis patients is β2-microglobulin and this is deposited within connective tissues and not in major organs.

48. NONE CORRECT

ACE inhibitors are relatively contraindicated in bilateral reno-vascular disease but they may be necessary for control of resulting hypertension; they may be useful in cases of unilateral renal artery stenosis. In IDDM, untreated renal failure is the commonest cause of death, whereas in NIDDM the majority of patients die from cardiovascular complications. Episodes of macroscopic haematuria in IgA nephropathy tend to occur at the same time as, or shortly after, an upper respiratory tract infection, and the majority of patients with reflux nephropathy have no relevant antecedent history. Although renal transplant function may be satisfactory after a period of cold ischaemia of up to 30 hours, donor organ warm ischaemia should be minimised and certainly should not exceed 45 minutes.

49. B D

Pulmonary fibrosis of silicosis and ankylosing spondylitis affects predominantly the upper zones whereas that of asbestosis, fibrosing alveolitis and systemic sclerosis occurs predominantly in the lower zones. In systemic sclerosis there may be a combination of diffuse fibrosis and basal aspiration pneumonia (see also Q.207 and Q.220).

50. A D

Perhaps the most important cause of pulmonary eosinophilia in the UK is allergic broncho-pulmonary aspergillosis. Other causes include allergic reactions to a variety of parasites such as filaria, (tropical eosinophilia) or drugs (nitrofurantoin, sulphonamides, chlorpropamide, and others). Loeffler's syndrome is a term used to describe mild transient illnesses with pulmonary eosinophilia for which no cause is found.

51. B C E

Muscle tone is at its lowest during REM sleep when complete obstruction tends to occur. Oximetry alone will show recurrent and persistent falls in oxygen saturation during periods of obstruction and is probably the best first line approach. A number of cardio-respiratory complications occur, including pulmonary arterial hypertension and cor pulmonale. Tracheostomy completely by-passes the obstruction and is almost 100% effective.

52. **C E**

Reactive arthritis may occur following enteric or urethral infections typically with Yersinia, Salmonella, Shigella, Campylobacter or Chlamydia. The joint is 'non-infective', enthesitis is common, hence the occurrence of tendonitis. Eye involvement is in the form of conjunctivitis or anterior uveitis (see also Q.226).

53. **A B C D**

Penicillamine can lower rheumatoid factor titres. The recorded side effects are legion: commonly rash and pruritus, ageusia (a blunting of taste perception which is not dose related), leucopenia, thrombo-cytopenia and proteinuria secondary to an immune complex nephritis. Rarer penicillamine-induced syndromes include myasthenia gravis, SLE, polymyositis, thyroiditis, haemolytic anaemia and Goodpasture's syndrome (see also Q.217 and Q.222).

54. **A B D E**

A number of conditions are desirable when carrying out a clinical trial of a new drug. Firstly, the drug should be safe and have been thoroughly tested in experimental animals. A pilot study is useful to help the design of the proper study, in particular to predict the number of observations required to attain a result of statistical significance. A double blind cross-over method is a well-tried and effective design, but is not uniformly applicable and can give rise to problems in certain circumstances. It is usually best to administer the drug to patients who are not undergoing treatment with other drugs as these may interfere with the results (see also Q.29).

55. **A C E**

Almost all patients taking lithium carbonate report polydipsia and polyuria, due to interference with ADH action in the kidney. A high serum lithium concentration causes gastro-intestinal disturb-ances, weakness and fine tremor of the hands, but not an intention tremor. There is a risk of hypothyroidism in patients taking lithium, due to effects on intrathyroid iodine metabolism.

56. A E

Atropine poisoning produces parasympathetic blockade and a toxic psychosis characterised by mania, hallucinations and delirium. There is dry mouth, dilated pupils, a dry, flushed skin, fever, tachycardia, urinary retention and abdominal distension. Atropine-like drugs used for Parkinsonism and gastro-intestinal disorders can give the same picture.

57. A B D E

Clinical parameters identified as indicating poor prognosis include severe hypotension (<75 mmHg systolic pressure), skin/rectal temperature difference of >3° C, Glasgow coma scale of <8, recent deterioration, absence of meningism and rapid extension of purpuric rash. Laboratory measures that are also helpful include the detection of meningococcal antigen in the serum and leucopenia.

58. A B C D E

Wheezing may result from endobronchial tuberculosis and this may be steroid responsive. In patients with disseminated/miliary tuberculosis, adult respiratory distress syndrome may occur and this tends to happen between one and three weeks after commencing antituberculous agents. Both pleural effusion and unilateral hilar lymphadenopathy are complications of primary tuberculosis. Remember that pleural effusion is a lymphocytic exudate with a low glucose ratio compared to blood, and a high adenosine deaminase level. Significant haemoptysis occurs in about 8%; massive haemoptysis (>1000 ml/24 h) can occur when there is erosion of a major blood vessel, either bronchial or pulmonary, and is a medical emergency. It is more common when there are cavities or bronchiectasis.

59. A B D E

Rat-bite fever can be due to two organisms – *Spirillum minis* which is a spirochaete and can be seen on blood films, and *Streptobacillus moniliformis* which is a fastidious Gram negative rod that is grown from blood cultures. *Borrelia recurrentis* is the cause of relapsing fever and is diagnosed by blood film examination whereas Lyme disease is caused by *Borrelia burgdorferi* and is diagnosed primarily by serology. Early African and American trypanosomiasis can be diagnosed by blood film as can Oroya fever, which is a bacterial infection of red cells caused by *Bartonella bacilliformis*. Of course the major reason for performing a blood film in patients with a fever recently returned from abroad is to diagnose malaria.

60. E

Jaundice is exceptionally rare in amoebic liver abscess unless the abscess is compressing one of the major intrahepatic bile ducts. Splenomegaly is also rarely seen and active concomitant dysentery only occurs in a minority of patients (15%) although about the same percentage will give a history of previous dysentery in the preceding 2 months. Only 1% of abscesses will rupture into the pericardium and these will be left lobe abscesses which only account for 1 in 5 of the total. This is the most serious complication and patients rapidly develop tamponade. A raised hemidiaphragm is commonly seen and is one of the most helpful radiological features (see also Q.120).

APPENDIX

INHERITED DISORDERS

1. The following are autosomal recessive conditions:

Albinism
Ataxia telangiectasia
Congenital adrenal hyperplasia
Crigler-Najjar syndrome type I
Cystic fibrosis
Deafness (some forms)
Dubin-Johnson syndrome
Fanconi's anaemia
Friedreich's ataxia
Galactosaemia
Gaucher's disease
Glycogen storage diseases

Haemochromatosis
Homocystinuria
Hurler's syndrome
Limb girdle muscular dystrophy
  (Erb)
Niemann-Pick disease
Phenylketonuria
Pendred's syndrome
Sickle cell disease
Thalassaemias
Tay-Sach's disease
Wilson's disease

2. The following are X-linked recessive, and therefore more common in males:

Agammaglobulinaemia
Becker's muscular dystrophy
Chronic granulomatous disease.
Complete testicular feminization
Duchenne muscular dystrophy
Fabry's disease
Glucose-6-phosphate dehydro-
  genase deficiency
Haemophilia A (VIII)

Haemophilia B (IX)
Hunter's syndrome
Ichthyosis
Lesch-Nyhan syndrome (hypox-
  anthine guanine phosphoribosyl
  transferase deficiency)
Nephrogenic diabetes insipidus
Ocular albinism
Wiskott-Aldrich syndrome

3. The following are autosomal dominant:

Achondroplasia
Acute intermittent porphyria
Adult polycystic kidney disease
Facioscapulohumeral dystrophy
Familial hypercholesterolaemia
Gilbert's syndrome
Huntington's chorea
Hereditary spherocytosis
Malignant hyperthermia
Marfan's syndrome

Myotonic dystrophy
Myotonia congenita
Neurofibromatosis
Noonan's syndrome
Osteogenesis imperfecta (some
  forms)
Polyposis coli
Rotor syndrome
Tuberose sclerosis
Von Willebrand's disease

MRCP PART I EXAMINATION: TOPIC DISTRIBUTION

A breakdown of the relative distribution of topics is given below.
Variations may occur from exam to exam.

Subject Area	Number of MCQs
Neurology	5/6
Clin. Pharmacology/Toxicology	5/6
Cardiology	4/5
Nephrology and electrolyte disorders	4/5
Basic Sciences	4/5
Gastroenterology	4
Respiratory Medicine	4
Infectious disease/AIDS/Tropical and GU medicine	4
Endocrinology	4
Rheumatology/Immunology	3/4
Paediatrics	3
Psychiatry	3
Haematology	3
Metabolic disorders	2
Dermatology	1
Statistics	1
Genetics	1
Ophthalmology	1
Total Number of MCQs	60

REVISION INDEX

Each item in this index refers to a specific reference contained in a question in this book. The numbers given are **question numbers** not page numbers and a number prefixed by p.ex indicates that the reference is to be found in the practice exam at the end of the book.